AF556367

AIDS EDUCATION TO COLLEGE STUDENTS

By

Dr. D. Sarada

&

Vijaya M. Udamala

DISCOVERY PUBLISHING HOUSE PVT. LTD.

NEW DELHI-110 002

First Published - 2009

Reprinted - 2017

ISBN: 978-81-8356-482-3

AIDS Education to College Students

Published by:

DISCOVERY PUBLISHING HOUSE PVT. LTD.

4383/4B, Ansari Road, Darya Ganj

New Delhi-110 002 (India)

Phone: +91-11-23279245, 43596064-65

Fax: +91-11-23253475

E-mail: discoverypublishinghouse@gmail.com

sales@discoverypublishinggroup.com

web: www.discoverypublishinggroup.com

Printed at:

Infinity Imaging Systems

Delhi

Acknowledgements

I owe my sincere gratitude to God Almighty, who accompanied and blessed me throughout this study. I express sincere thanks to all those without whose contribution this project would not have been possible.

The present study has been completed under the guidance of Dr. D. Sarada, Professor, Department of Home Science (Human Development and Family Studies), Sri Padmavathi Mahila Visvavidyalayam, Tirupati. I wholeheartedly express my sincere gratitude to Dr. D. Sarada for her enduring patience, inspiration, constant support, encouragement and valuable suggestions from the inception to the completion of the study. I consider it a great privilege to work under her expert guidance.

I am grateful to Dr. A. Violet. Professor and Dr. E. Manjuvani, Professor SPMVV for their valuable suggestions. I am also thankful to Dr. Rajeswari, the Librarian and Library staff SPMVV College Library for helping to utilise the library facilities. I owe my sincere gratitude to the Head and the staff of the Department of Home Science for their administrative support. I am grateful to all the experts for validating the data collection instruments and education programme.

I am highly indebted to Rev. Sr. Theresia Supriyati, Superior General and General Council Sr. Pia de Ridder (Late), Sr. Regina and Sr. Fabiola of the Soc. of JMJ, The Netherlands and Rev. Stella Maris, Provincial Superior,

Sr. Regis, Sr. Emily, Sr. Showrilu Provincial Council, Guntur Province for their constant support and encouragement.

My cordial thanks to Sr. Innamma and Council, Hyderabad Province and Sr. Lillian and Council, Bangalore Province and all the sisters of JMJ for their prayers and support throughout my study.

I am grateful to the principals and faculty of Junior colleges for extending their help in the conduct of the study. I am indebted to all the students of junior colleges for extending their co-operation without which it would have been impossible to conduct the study.

My heartfelt thanks to Sr. Gladys Inviolata, the Principal, and the faculty of St. Joseph's College of Nursing and Sr. Roseline, the Office Manager for their concern and help in the conduct of the study. My appreciation and gratitude to Siva, Lakshmi and Bala who helped me with numerous requests during the study period.

A word of commendation to Siva Nageswara Rao and Chandra Sekhar Reddy for typing and printing the manuscript and Mr. Lingaiah, the Statistician for his guidance in statistical analysis. A word of appreciation to Mrs. Deva Krupa for editing the manuscript.

I am deeply grateful to Sr. Manjula and Sr. Saritha for their timely assistance in the development and editing of the video film on crusade against AIDS. My heartfelt gratitude to Sr. Vijaya S for her valuable suggestions and help.

I extend my hearty thanks to my beloved family and friends for their constant encouragement and support.

Vijaya M Udamala

Foreword

HIV/AIDS still remains a threat to development of people of all ages and Nationalities. It is pandemic, now at the beginning of its third decade, is one of the most devastating diseases, currently. It deprives families, communities and entire nations of people at their most productive ages. This epidemic is deepening poverty, affecting human development achievements, worsening gender inequalities, and eroding the ability of governments to maintain essential services, reducing labour Productivity, supply, and hampering economic growth in the Countries worst affected for decades to come (UNAIDS, 2005).

It is alarming to note that 40.3 million adults and 2.5 million children were living with HIV (UNAIDS, 2005) at the end of 2005. Around half of all people who become infected with HIV do so before they are 25 years and are killed by AIDS, before they are 35 years thus wasting human resource. Deaths among those already infected will continue to increase for some years even if prevention programmes manage to cut the number of new infections to zero. However, with the HIV positive population still expanding the annual no. of AIDS deaths and expected to increase for many years.

Young people (15-24 years) account for half of all new HIV infections world wide, and more than Rs. 6,00,000 become infected with HIV every year. After 25 years, people are still making resources and plans on how to address the epidemic when there is no need any more. People have been dying for the past two and half decades and there are innumerable resources, available already.

Some forms of Aids education have been shown to be more effective than others, but what is essentially important is that the population is informed about the damages and made known how to protect themselves and others. Several innovative programmes have been organized to create awareness and fear appeal to the public and high-risk population to protect them. As quoted the World Bank (2004) by the author, it is necessary to reinforce that "AIDS education is a social vaccine to protect people from getting infected. Education is one of the most effective and cost effective HIV preventive strategies. Education has strong potential to make a difference in the sight against HIV/AIDS". Even in UK and USA, still there is stigma on and discrimination of AIDS affected population. However it is not surprising to note that it is persistent in India. Care and support model is one of the best models in the world. It is in this context, the author made a sincere and scientific attempt to educate adolescent girls to protect themselves and others from AIDS. This publication can serve as a resource to guide governments, education and health authorities, advisers, educational institutions, teachers, health care persons and trainers in improving the sex/AIDS education and ensuring it meets the needs of young youth. The interest in effectiveness reflects the trends towards evidence based and demonstrable outcomes in education. In addition to publication, researchers need to tap the opportunities to join the advisors, trainers and practitioners to share the findings of the implementation of AIDS education and to consider its implications for further development of effective strategies to AIDS education. This will go a long was in preventing AIDS infection during productive years of the population and thus contributing to economic growth of the nations directly or indirectly.

Prof. K. Chandralekha
Former Dean & Registrar,
Sri Padmavati Mahila Visva Vidyalayam,
Tirupati

Contents

1 Introduction

HIV still remains a threat to people of all ages and nationalities.

"Education is a Social Vaccine to protect people from getting infected. Education is one of the most effective and cost effective HIV preventive strategies. Education has strong potential to make a difference in the fight against HIV/AIDS.."

—World Bank, 2004

After 25 years, people are still making resources and plans on how to address the epidemic when there is no need anymore. People have been dying for the past two and half decades and there are innumerable resources available already. Some forms of AIDS education have been shown to be more effective than others, but what is essentially important is that the population is informed about the dangers and made known how to protect themselves and other people.

According to UNAIDS (2005) estimates there were 40.3 million adults and 2.5 million children living with HIV at the end of 2005. Around half of all people who become infected with HIV do so before they are twenty five years and are killed by AIDS before they are thirty five years. During 2005, some five million people became infected with the human immunodeficiency virus (HIV), which causes AIDS. The year also saw 3.1 million deaths from HIV/AIDS, a high global total, despite antiretroviral therapy, which reduced AIDS and AIDS related deaths in the richer countries. Deaths among those already infected will continue to increase for some years even if prevention programmes manage to cut the number of new infections to zero. However, with the HIV positive population still expanding the annual number of AIDS deaths can be expected to increase for many years (UNAIDS /WHO Epidemic update, 2005).

More than 25 million people have died of AIDS since 1981. Africa has 12 million orphans. By December 2005 women accounted for 46 per cent of all adults living with HIV worldwide, and for 57 per cent in sub-Saharan Africa. By the end of 2005, the epidemic has left behind a cumulative total of 15 million AIDS Orphans, defined as those having lost one or both parents to AIDS before reaching the age of fifteen years.

Young people (15-24 years old) account for half of all new HIV infections worldwide, and more than 6,00,000 become infected with HIV every year. In 2005, an estimated 7,00,000 children aged fourteen or younger became infected with HIV. Over 90 per cent were born to HIV-positive women, who acquired the virus at birth or through their mother's breast milk.

Of the overwhelming majority of people with HIV, some 95 per cent of the global total, live in the developing world. The proportion is set to grow even further as infection rates continue to rise in countries where poverty, poor health care systems and limited resources for prevention and care fuel the spread of the virus.

In the future, every human service worker will be in contact with an individual with HIV/AIDS. The rate of confirmed cases is rising in alarming numbers. According to All, Juliet and Roberto (1993) no other medical event in recent history has produced the amount of public fear and private response as the AIDS epidemic. This fear may well be the driving force behind all behavioural responses to AIDS.

HIV/AIDS has been thought of in the past as a disease mainly affecting high-risk groups like gay men or drug users. In fact in 2005, 85 per cent of HIV infections are due to heterosexual sex, women are more likely to be infected than men.

Across India today, HIV/AIDS is seen to be moving from high-risk groups to the more vulnerable segments among the general population. It is generally thought that HIV first appeared in the northeast states amongst intravenous drug users. However, the first serological evidence of HIV infection in India was found in 1986, from among female sex workers in Tamil Nadu. Through the eighties, nineties and the first five years of the new millennium, HIV has been detected in a range of population groups and locations. We know that HIV has spread from 1.75 million people infected in 1994 to 5.134 million in people in 2004, across all states and union territories in India. In India the adult prevalence rate is about 0.9 per cent. India accounts for 10 per cent of global HIV burden and 65 per cent of that in South and South East Asia. (NACO, 2004)

The AIDS pandemic, now at the beginning of its third decade, is one of the most devastating diseases of our time. Concerted national and international efforts are needed to prevent the spread of HIV and to break the silence that still continues to surround the disease in many countries. The disaster caused by HIV/AIDS is unique because it deprives families, communities and entire nations of people at their most productive ages. The epidemic is deepening poverty, reversing human development achievements, worsening gender inequalities, eroding the ability of governments to maintain essential services, reducing labour productivity and supply and hampering economic growth in the countries worst affected for decades to come. (UNAIDS, 2005).

NEED FOR THE STUDY

Nurses and midwives are in a unique position by virtue of their education, numbers, and diversity of practice arenas to contribute to the health of adolescents. In collaboration with the WHO Departments of Human Resources for Health, the core competencies were developed for professional nursing and midwifery education worldwide. It also includes strategies for integrating adolescent health and development into curricula and several tools to assist in this integration. These include the right to: non-discrimination, education and access to appropriate information, privacy and confidentiality, protection from all forms of violence, rest, leisure and play, an adequate standard of living, freedom from all forms of exploitation, participation, including the right to be heard.

In order for adolescents to take the risks that are important for their development and avoid those that will do them irreparable harm, their rights to health and development need to be fulfilled. This includes their rights to information and skills, a range of services, a safe and supportive environment, and opportunities to participate. Frequently, this is not the case. HIV/AIDS flourishes where human rights are not protected.

Adolescents are vulnerable because they often do not know how serious the problem of HIV/AIDS is, how it is caused or what they can do to protect themselves. Many adolescents do not go to school, and do not have access to information about AIDS, or to opportunities to develop the life skills that they need to turn this information into action. Frequently they also do not have access to services that take their specific needs into consideration.

In addition to the individual characteristics of young people themselves, they are also influenced by other young people and made vulnerable by the attitudes and behaviours of the significant adults in their lives, such as parents, teachers and service providers. The wider context in which they live, learn and work, including social values and norms, policies and legislation, and their economic situation are also very important.

Some young people are particularly vulnerable. In countries where the predominant mode of transmission is by heterosexual sex, girls are often more vulnerable than boys, for both biological and social reasons. Young people involved with sex work, migrants and refugees, and adolescents living on the street, in war situations or who are marginalised and discriminated against, are all likely to be especially vulnerable. Of course vulnerability is also increased by HIV/AIDS itself, for example young people who are living with HIV/AIDS and AIDS orphans (of whom large proportions are adolescents) become even more vulnerable to HIV/AIDS.

Young People—a window of hope in the HIV/AIDS pandemic. The HIV/AIDS pandemic is one of the most important and urgent public health challenges facing governments and civil societies around the world. Adolescents are at the centre of the pandemic in terms of transmission, impact, and potential for changing the attitudes and behaviours that underlies this disease. It is estimated that 50 per cent of all new HIV infections are among young people (about 7,000 young people become infected every day), and that 30 per cent of the 40 million people living with HIV/AIDS are in the 15-24 year age group. The vast majority of young people who are HIV positive do not know that they are infected, and few young people who are engaging in sex know the HIV status of their partners.

The importance of focussing on young people has been recognised at a global level by the 2001 UN General Assembly Special Session on HIV/AIDS, which endorsed a number of goals for young people, including: By 2003, establish time-bound national targets to achieve the internationally agreed global prevention goal to reduce by 2005 HIV prevalence among young men and women aged 15-24 years in the most affected countries by 25 per cent and by 25 per cent globally by 2010. By 2005, ensure that at least 90 per cent, and by 2010 at least 95 per cent of young men and women have access to the information, education, including peer education and youth-specific education, and services necessary to develop the life skills required to reduce their vulnerability to HIV infection; in full partnership with youth, parents, families, educators and health care providers.

Focussing on young people is likely to be the most effective approach to confronting the epidemic, particularly in high prevalence countries. In March 2003, WHO organised a global consultation, in collaboration with UNAIDS, UNFPA, UNICEF and Youth Net, on the health services response to the prevention and care of HIV/AIDS among young people. Protecting young people from HIV and AIDS publication, on the role of health services is based on the outcome of this consultation, and has been developed for a wide readership of policy makers and programmers. The publication provides an overview of the evidence on health service interventions that are important for achieving the global goals on young people and HIV/AIDS: information and counselling reducing risk through condoms and harm reduction; and the diagnosis, treatment and care of STIs and HIV/AIDS. In addition, it describes key strategies for delivering these interventions, outlines the quality characteristics of effective health services for young people, and identifies issues that will need to be taken into consideration when developing national targets for measuring progress towards achieving the goals.

Each year an estimated 333 million new cases of curable sexually transmitted infections (STI) occur worldwide with the highest rates among 20-24 year olds, followed by 15-19 year olds. One in 20 young people are believed to contract a STI each year, excluding HIV and other viral infections. A minority of adolescents has access to any acceptable and affordable STI services.

A veteran AIDS expert has warned that India has raced to the top position with the largest number of people carrying the deadly HIV, much more than South Africa. Richard Feachem, in-charge of malaria, tuberculosis and HIV at The Global Fund, one of the largest AIDS donors said in an interview in Paris that figures are much higher than those given by the Government of India. Feachem said that his is a wake up call as the government is not doing enough and millions might die due to the delay. (UNAIDS, 2005)

The Indian government is also criticised for clinging to the idea that the epidemic is limited to "high risk groups", such as sex workers, drug users and truck drivers and that targeting them is the best strategy to contain the epidemic further. But this approach no longer reflects the reality of at least some Indian states, where the epidemic is in the general population. In these states women who only have sex with their husbands may be the group at highest risk of HIV transmission, and although in Indian society men can experiment with sex outside of marriage, women do not have status to demand condom use of their husbands.

Comprehensive AIDS education can make pupils aware of the need to protect themselves against infection. It can also bring about gradual changes in the wider social environment, making safer sex more acceptable. Educating people about HIV/AIDS and prevention is complicated as India has many major languages and hundreds of different dialects. So although some HIV/AIDS prevention and education can be done at the national level many of the efforts are best carried out at the state and local level.

"Women and AIDS" is the theme of the 2004 World AIDS day. In many parts of the world, discrimination prevents people who are known to have HIV from securing a job or caring for their families. Discrimination can cause isolation and marginalizes people who have HIV and AIDS. This can prevent people from being offered or seeking the treatment, which could save their lives. In order of HIV to be effectively tackled on an international level, efforts need to be made to end the discrimination against people with HIV and AIDS, educate people in safer sex and drug use, using appropriate media, provide condoms freely to people in the developing world, provide financial and medical assistance so that people with HIV and AIDS can be treated.

According to the UNAIDS what is needed on a massive national and international level is to:

- End the stifling silence that continues to surround HIV in many countries.
- Explode myths and misconceptions that translate into dangerous sexual practices.

- ❖ Expand prevention initiatives such as condom promotion that can reduce sexual transmission.
- ❖ Create conditions in which young children have the knowledge and the emotional and financial support to grow up free of HIV.
- ❖ Devote real money for providing care for those infected with HIV and support to their families.
- ❖ A trail of successful responses has already been blased by a small number of dedicated communities and governments. The challenge for everyone is to adapt and massively expand successful approaches that make it harder for the virus to spread, and that make it easier for those affected to live full and rewarding lives. (WHO, 2005)

Each year there are more and more new HIV infections. This shows that people either aren't learning the message about the dangers of HIV, or are unable or unwilling to act on it. Many people are dangerously ignorant about the virus—a survey in the UK found recently that a third of teens thought there was a 'cure' for AIDS. Education is an important component of preventing the spread of HIV. Even if education were completely successful, it would still have to be an ongoing process—each generation a new generation of people become adult and need to know how to protect them from infection. The older generations, who have hopefully already been educated, may need the message reinforced, and need to be kept informed, so that they are able to protect themselves and inform the younger.

There are two main reasons for AIDS education, the first of which is to prevent new infections. This can be seen as consisting of two processes:

- ❖ Giving people information about HIV—what HIV and AIDS are how they are transmitted and how people can protect them from infection.
- ❖ Teaching people how to put this information to use and act on it practically how to get and use condoms,

how to suggest and practice safer sex, how to prevent infection in a medical environment or when injecting drugs.

The second reason people need AIDS education is to reduce stigma and discrimination. In many countries there is a great deal of fear and stigmatisation of people who are HIV positive. Ignorance, resentment and ultimately, anger too often accompany this fear. Sometimes the results of prejudice and fear can be extreme, with HIV positive people being burned to death in India, and many families being forced to leave their homes across the United States when neighbours discover a family-member's positive status. Discrimination against positive people can help the AIDS epidemic to spread—if people are fearful of being tested for HIV, and then they are more likely to pass the infection to someone else without knowing.

Anyone who is vulnerable to AIDS and almost everyone is vulnerable, unless they know how to protect themselves. It's not only young people, injecting drug users or gay men who become infected—the virus has affected a cross-section of society needs to be educated. This means that education ought to be aimed at all parts of society, not only those groups who are seen as being particularly high-risk.

If AIDS education that had been done up until now had been fully effective, then there wouldn't have been five million new infections in 2005. It is clear that the campaigns carried out so far have failed to prevent the spread of the virus, so the message needs to be repeated, in different forms, until people appreciate it, or until, hopefully, education is no longer needed.

AIDS education doesn't always take place in a classroom. It can be presented in many ways and put across by many forms of media, which should be selected with the target group in mind. Some people can be best reached via newspapers and magazines, whilst other people might be more used to street theatre as a form of media. AIDS education needs to embrace culturally appropriate and relevant media. These might include radio, television, billboard advertising, street theatre, comic strips, etc. Sometimes AIDS education is about giving people information which they will remember on a long term basis, about how to protect themselves, the difference between HIV and AIDS, and helping to reduce discrimination. On other occasions, an education strategy might intend to have a more immediate effect and target people when they are most likely to take part in risky behaviour.

There are a number of different methods, which can be used to educate the public about the dangers of HIV. Peer education is, quite simply, a social form of education without classrooms or notebooks, where people are educated outside a 'school' environment but still have the opportunity to ask questions. Sometimes the 'peer educators' will be from the group that is to be educated—a group of workmates might pick someone from amongst them to become the educator. Only other occasions the educator may be someone who has a similar social background, age and gender to the target audience, sometimes a person who is HIV+. Most peer education focuses on providing information about HIV transmission and answering questions. The sessions take place wherever it is convenient, sometimes in Schools/ Colleges, workplace or where a group of women gather to wash clothes.

Education is an important part of AIDS prevention, but it is only one part. AIDS prevention work being done around the world covers such diverse topics as the search for a vaccine, distribution of condoms, research into microbicides, lobbying governmental organisations, and testing people to monitor the trends of the epidemic. Education, however, is a crucial factor in preventing the spread of HIV, and, given the huge numbers of deaths that might still be prevented; the importance of effective education cannot be overestimated.

Although the debate continues about how much, AIDS education young people should receive, studies continue to show that being informed about the facts and the dangers of HIV/AIDS enables young people to protect themselves and is a crucial tool in the battle against HIV. There is no cure or vaccine for HIV, prevention is the only way in which we can place any limits on the epidemic. One of the most economical and effective means of HIV prevention is education, involving young people themselves in the HIV prevention effort.

Although the AIDS epidemic is well into its third decade, basic AIDS education remains fundamental to the global effort to prevent HIV transmission. AIDS education can and does target all ages, and sexually active adults are one principal target. AIDS education is also vitally important for young people, however, and Schools/Colleges offer a crucial point-of-contact for their receiving this education.

The World AIDS Campaign's theme for 2005 is "Stop AIDS: Keep the Promise". This theme is however not specific to World AIDS Day alone but it will also remain the focus until 2010. "Stop AIDS. Keep the Promise" is an appeal to governments and policy makers to ensure they meet the targets they have agreed to in the fight against HIV and AIDS. Some of the most important of these promises are contained in the UN Declaration of Commitment, which was signed by all 189 members of the UN in June 2001. The governments of these countries committed themselves to take action on HIV and AIDS in the fields of leadership, prevention, care and support, treatment, reducing vulnerability, and human rights. The following targets were set for the end of 2005:

- Reduce HIV prevalence by 25 per cent among men and women aged 15-24 in the most affected countries.
- Ensure that at least 90 per cent of young people aged 15 to 24 have access to the information, education and services necessary to develop the life skills required to reduce their vulnerability to HIV infection.

- ❖ Reduce the proportion of infants infected with HIV by 20 per cent by increasing access to services, which prevent mother-to-child transmission.
- ❖ Increase annual spending on HIV and AIDS to $7-10 billion in low and middle-income countries and those countries experiencing or at risk of experiencing rapid expansion of HIV epidemics.

People have a right to hold governments and policy makers to account as they announce whether these promises have been kept, and whether enough progress is being made towards longer-term targets.

The epidemic of HIV has been steadily spreading for the past more than two decades and now affects every country in the world. Each year, more people die, and the number of people living with HIV continues to rise, in spite of the fact that we have developed many proven HIV prevention methods. One of the key means of HIV prevention is education, teaching people about HIV: what it is, what it does, and how people can protect themselves. Over half of the world's population is now under 25 years old, and they are both the age group most threatened by AIDS and the best hope of combating the epidemic. Education can help to fight HIV, and it must focus on young people.

Despite women's higher biological vulnerability, it is the legal, social and economic disadvantages faced by women and girls in most societies that greatly increase their HIV vulnerability. Therefore, gender sensitive approaches are key issues, when designing prevention programmes. (WHO, 2003)

Many women are denied the knowledge and tools to protect themselves from HIV. Surveys in 38 countries found extremely low HIV-transmission knowledge among 15-24 year old women (UNFPA, 2002). It is vital to implement comprehensive strategies, including gender-specific and culturally specific services that help women counteract discriminatory social and economic factors. Key components include: access to education (particularly secondary education); strengthening legal protection for women's property and inheritance rights; eradicating violence against women and girls; and ensuring equitable access to HIV care and prevention services.

In June 2002, the World Health Organisation and the International Center for Research on Women led a consultation of experts to rethink classic HIV prevention based on women's and girls' distinct needs. They also aimed to improve HIV interventions that target men. Gender-sensitive approaches, at a minimum, recognise that women and men have different prevention, care and support needs. For example, diagnosing and treating sexually transmitted infections need to be integrated into family planning/reproductive health clinics. Then women will be able to gain access to these services without fear of social censure. (WHO, 2003)

Interventions that empower women and girls attempt to equalize the power balance between women and men. Examples include increasing women's access to assets and resources, such as land and inheritance rights, and facilitating women's networks and strengthening grassroots community organisations. Other projects go beyond immediate gender-specific needs. They are based on the belief that empowerment can only be achieved when women take control of all aspects of their lives.

Although the epidemic is well spread into its third decade, basic AIDS education remains fundamental to the response. For instance, in India, behavioural survey data showed that 30 per cent of women had not heard of HIV or AIDS Rural women were the least informed: less than 25 per cent of rural women in the states of Bihar (18.7 per cent), Gujarat (22.7 per cent) and Uttar Pradesh (24.3 per cent) were aware that HIV could be transmitted sexually. (NACO, 2003)

In 1987 in the UK, a leaflet about AIDS was delivered to every household, and the government also launched a major advertising campaign with the slogan *"AIDS: Don't Die of*

Ignorance." Ignorance is not bliss. Ignorance costs lives. No one deserves to get AIDS. Everyone has right to proper information, education and communication about HIV/AIDS.

Young Girls during their adolescent period are often particularly vulnerable to sexually transmitted HIV, and to HIV infection as a result of drug-use. Studies have proved that Young people (15-24 years old) account for half of all new HIV infections worldwide and more than 6,000 become infected with HIV every day. More than a third of all people living with HIV or AIDS are under the age of twenty five years and almost two-thirds of them are women (NACO, 2005).

In many parts of the world, young people in this age group are at particularly high risk of HIV infection from unprotected sex. Indeed, globally, most young people become sexually active in their teens. The fact that they are or soon will be at risk of HIV infection makes young people a crucial target for AIDS education.

With 75.73 million population as on the 2001 censes, Andhra Pradesh is India's fifth most populous state in the country. It is also on the country's six high HIV/AIDS prevalence states. Based on the sentinel surveillance data, it is estimated by NACO (2004) that over 51,53,221 are infected with HIV in India and almost one tenth i.e. 5,00,000 above infections are in Andhra Pradesh. HIV prevalence varies substantially across the districts of Andhra Pradesh. In 12 of the state's 23 districts, more than 2 per cent of women attending antenatal clinics tested positive for HIV in 2004. Most of these districts are in Costal Andhra Pradesh. (APSACS, 2005)

Guntur one among the coastal districts is confronted with high prevalence rates of HIV infection not only among High risk groups but also among general population. Young Girls during their adolescent period are often particularly vulnerable to sexually transmitted HIV, and to HIV infection as a result of drug-use. The fact that they are or soon will be at risk of HIV infection makes young people a crucial target for AIDS education.

HIV/AIDS awareness needs to be reinforced among the students right from school to college levels. College is a good platform as the students at this level are to understand themselves well and teacher is the most authentic person to pass on the information to students on HIV/AIDS. Just adding a chapter in the syllabi will not better the situation. What is more important is making the youngsters feel responsible for their behaviour and life style. (Damayanthi, Project Director, APSACS 2004)

Several innovative programmes have been implemented to create awareness among general public as well as high risk population. School and College based AIDS education programme has been organised by Government and non government organisations encouraging students to adopt positive life styles required for prevention of HIV/AIDS. Often such efforts have become sporadic than regular feature in the schools and colleges. Hence, the present study is a felt necessity to impart HIV/AIDS information to adolescent girls who have a great potential to learn and increase their knowledge, develop positive attitude and favourable practice regarding HIV/AIDS and also to reach out to their peers, families and the society at large with AIDS awareness message.

STATEMENT OF THE PROBLEM

A Study to Evaluate the Effectiveness of an AIDS Education Programme to Adolescent Girls of Junior Colleges in Guntur District of Andhra Pradesh.

AIM OF THE STUDY

To impart HIV/AIDS Education to the adolescent girls and evaluate its impact on their knowledge, attitude and practice regarding HIV/AIDS.

OBJECTIVES OF THE STUDY

1. To develop tools for assessing the Knowledge, Attitude and Practice of the adolescent girls on HIV/AIDS.
2. To develop and validate AIDS Education Programme (AEP).

3. To develop AIDS Education Programme manual in print and electronic multi media for AIDS Education.
4. To assess the Knowledge, Attitude and Practice of the adolescent girls of Junior Colleges on HIV/AIDS before and after the administration of AIDS Education Programme.
5. To study the effectiveness of the AIDS Education Programme in terms of gains in Knowledge, Attitude, and Practice among the adolescent girls of Junior Colleges.
6. To study the relationship between Knowledge, Attitude and Practice of adolescent girls on HIV/ AIDS.
7. To study the association between independent variables such as Age, Year of Study, Religion, Caste, Place of Residence, Type of Family, Family Income and dependent variables Knowledge, Attitude and Practice.

HYPOTHESES

H_1 The mean post-test I Knowledge scores of Junior College Students exposed to AEP will be significantly higher than their mean pre-test Knowledge scores as measured by Knowledge scale at 0.05 level of significance.

H_2 The mean post-test I Attitude scores of Junior College Students exposed to AEP will be significantly higher than their mean pre-test Attitude scores as measured by Attitude scale at 0.05 level of significance.

H_3 The mean post-test I Practice scores of Junior College Students exposed to AEP will be significantly higher than that of their mean pre-test Practice scores as measured by Practice scale at 0.05 level of significance.

H_4 The mean gain in Knowledge score of Junior College Students exposed to AEP will be significantly higher than the mean gain in Knowledge scores of those who are not exposed to AEP as measured by Knowledge scale at 0.05 level of significance.

H_5 The mean gain in Attitude score of Junior college students exposed to AEP will be significantly higher than the mean gain in Attitude scores of those who are not exposed to AEP as measured by Attitude scale at 0.05 level of significance.

H_6 The mean gain in Practice score of Junior college students exposed to AEP will be significantly higher than the mean gain in Practice scores of those who are not exposed to AEP as measured by Practice scale at 0.05 level of significance.

H_7 There will be a significant relationship between Knowledge and Attitude scores of Junior college students before and after the administration of AEP regarding HIV/AIDS as evident from Knowledge and Attitude scores at 0.05 level of significance.

H_8 There will be a significant relationship between Knowledge and Practice scores of Junior college students before and after the administration of AEP regarding HIV/AIDS as evident from Knowledge and Practice scores at 0.05 level of significance.

H_9 There will be a significant relationship between Attitude and Practice scores of Junior college students before and after the administration of AEP regarding HIV/AIDS as evident from Attitude and Practice scores at 0.05 level of significance.

H_{10} There will be a significant relationship between Knowledge and Attitude Knowledge and Practice, Attitude and Practice post-test II scores of Junior college students regarding HIV/AIDS as evident from KAP post-test II scores at 0.05 level of significance.

H_{11} There will be a significant relationship between post-test I and post-test II Knowledge, Attitude and Practice scores of Junior college students regarding HIV/AIDS as evident from KAP post-test I and post-test II scores at 0.05 level of significance.

H_{12} There will be a significant association between the selected independent variables: Age, Year of Study,

Place of Residence, Religion, Caste, Type of Family, Family Income, and dependent variable Knowledge at 0.05 level of significance.

H_{13} There will be a significant association between the selected independent variables: Age, Year of Study, Place of residence, Religion, Caste, Type of family, Family income, and dependent variable Attitude at 0.05 level of significance.

H_{14} There will be a significant association between the selected independent variables: Age, Year of Study, Place of Residence, Religion, Caste, Type of Family, Family Income, and dependent variable Practice at 0.05 level of significance.

H_{15} There will be a significant contribution of Knowledge test scores to Attitude and Practice test scores at 0.05 level of significance.

SUMMARY OF THE CHAPTER

This chapter dealt with the introduction, need for study, and statement of the problem, aim of the study, objectives and the hypotheses of the study.

2 Review of Literature

Researchers almost never conduct a study in an intellectual vacuum; their studies are usually undertaken within the context of an existing knowledge base. One of the major functions of a research literature review is to ascertain what is already known in relation to a problem of interest (Polit & Hungler, 1999).

The review of related literature for the present study has been organised under the following headings:

HIV/AIDS; Concept and Definition.

Overview of the Global HIV/AIDS Epidemic.

HIV/AIDS and India's Response.

HIV/AIDS and Andhra Pradesh State's Response.

Historical Perspective of HIV/AIDS Research.

Youth / Adolescents and HIV/AIDS.

Knowledge, Attitude and Practice of Women and Adolescent Girls regarding HIV/AIDS.

Prevention and Control of HIV/AIDS and the Role of the Family, Society, Government and Non Government Organisations.

HIV/AIDS Education Programmes/Strategies and Methodologies used for HIV/AIDS Education.

HIV/AIDS—CONCEPT AND DEFINITION

No one knows exactly where the Human Immunodeficiency Virus originated, or the conditions that led to its spread among humans in the early 1980s. HIV-1 was identified in 1983 by Dr. Robert Gallo and other medical scientists at the National Cancer Institute in Bethesda, Maryland. At about the same time, Dr. Luc Montagnier of the Pasteur Institute in Paris isolated HIV-2 from AIDS patients. These two HIV viruses are distinguishable by their genome make up today, but are believed to have had a common ancestor in Africa. (Singhal & Rogers, 2003)

The first cases of AIDS were diagnosed in 1981. Some physicians in California and New York came across unusual opportunistic infections among homosexual men. These infections did not respond to medication. Therefore, the patients could not live longer and eventually died. These patients did not show usual conditions of illness known to Medical Science at that time. Thus, it became evident that we have a new illness to be treated. This new disease was named: "Acquired Immuno-deficiency Syndrome" (AIDS).

The HIV (Human Immuno-deficiency Virus) is a unique virus, very small and fragile. It can not survive outside the human body. HIV is a member of a group of viruses called Retroviruses. The virus enters the Helper T-cells of the immune system. In the helper T-cells it destroys genetic material and the damage caused is permanent. Thus, HIV hinders our immune system from protecting our body. Once HIV has attacked our immune system, our defense system becomes weakened. Since the body's immune system is weakened with the absence of helper T-cells, opportunistic infections attack the human body. People with HIV thus will stay sick althrough and die eventually. All body fluids contain helper T-cells. The concentration is high in blood, semen and vaginal secretion. (WHO SEARO No: 26)

HIV was first identified as "Lymphadenopathy Associated Virus" by the French Scientists and Virus III by the researchers of USA and the present name that is HIV was given in May

1986 by International committee on taxonomy. Both HIV-1 and HIV- 2 are found in India, although the majority of infections (91 per cent) are from HIV- 1, subtype C. HIV in India is overwhelmingly transmitted heterosexually. The three other known routes of transmission are through contaminated blood, use of unsterilised syringes and needles by injecting drug users, and perinatal transmission.

The word "virus" is Latin for "poison" an appropriate name for HIV, since no cure exists for it. The HIV which is so small that 16,000 can sit on the head of a pin, invades a living white blood cell, and reIit to reproduce the virus. One HIV virus can make an astounding 10 billion copies of itself in a day, with a mutation rate of 1 in 10,000. This notorious rate of random mutation can make HIV resistant to drugs. The rapid mutation also makes the development of a vaccine very difficult. The HIV infects a type of white blood cells known as T lymphocytes, also called T helper cells. They protect the human body against infections. The CD4 cells count measures the strength of an individual's immune system. A healthy adult has between 700 to 1,500 CD4 cells per cubic milliliter of blood. Over a period of years the T cell count of an HIV positive individual drops to a critical level, below 500, a sign of a depressed immune system. Below 200, the individual usually develops opportunistic infections. (Singhal and Rogers, 2003)

Acquire Immuno-deficiency Syndrome (AIDS) is a serious illness and public health crisis that merits the concerns of everyone. AIDS, which is one of the most dreaded diseases of humanity, has spread to every part of the world, threatening people from all spheres of life. The first case of HIV infection was reported in 1981 among the homosexuals in the United States of America, while HIV was first reported in India, in 1986 among the commercial sex workers from Chennai.

OVERVIEW OF THE GLOBAL HIV/AIDS EPIDEMIC

WHO and UNAIDS estimate that at the end of 2005, 40.3 Million people around the world were living with HIV. The epidemic is now spreading rapidly in Asia, where new infections are increasing faster than anywhere else in the world.

Table 2.1: Global Estimates of the HIV/AIDS Epidemic, as of end 2005

		Estimate	*Range*
People newly infected with HIV in 2005	Total	4.9 Million	(4.3- 6.6 Million)
	Adults	4.2 Million	(3.6 - 5.8 Million)
	Children < 15 years	0.70	(0.63-0.82)
Number of people living with HIV/AIDS in 2005	Total	40.3 Million	(34.5-42.6 Million)
	Adults	38 Million	(34.5 - 42.6 Million)
	Children < 15 years	2.3 Million	(2.1 - 2.8 Million)
AIDS deaths in 2005	Total	3.1 Million	(2.8- 3.6 Million)
	Adults	2.6 Million	(2.3 -2.9 Million)
	Children < 15 years	0.57 Million	(0.51-0.67 Million)
Total no. of AIDS death since the beginning of the epidemic until the end of 2005	Total	25 Million	
Total no. of the AIDS orphans since the beginning of the epidemic until the end of 2005	Total	15 Million	

Source: UNAIDS /WHO AIDS Epidemic Update, 2005.

In Africa south of the Sahara desert, an estimated 3.2 million adults and children became infected with HIV during the year 2005. This brought the total number of people living with HIV/AIDS in the region to 25.8 million by the end of the year.

For the moment, overall HIV prevalence, the regional total of people living with HIV or AIDS continues to rise because there are still more newly infected individuals joining it every year than there are people leaving it through death. However, as people infected years ago succumb to HIV related illnesses (average survival in absence of antiretroviral therapy is estimated at around 8-10 years), mortality from AIDS is increasing. HIV prevalence varies considerably across the continent—ranging from less than 1 per cent in Mauritania to almost 40 per cent in Botswana and Swaziland.

The AIDS epidemic in Eastern Europe and Central Asia shows no signs of declining. Some 2,70,000 people were infected with HIV in 2005, bringing the total number of people living with the virus to 1.6 million. AIDS claimed 62,000 lives in the past year. Worst affected are the Russian Federation, Ukraine, and the Baltic States (Estonia, Latvia, and Lithuania), but HIV continues to spread in Belarus, Moldova and Kazakhstan, while more recent epidemics are now evident in Kyrgyzstan and Uzbekistan. It is now estimated that around 1 million people aged 15-49 are living with HIV in the Russian Federation. Over 1 million people in Asia and the Pacific acquired HIV in 2005, bringing the number of people living with HIV to an estimated 7.4 million. A further 5,00,000 people are estimated to have died of AIDS in 2005.

In the North Africa and Middle East region 51,000 people acquired HIV infection in 2005, bringing the total number of people living with HIV/AIDS in the Middle East and North Africa to 6,00,000. AIDS killed a further 58,000 people in 2005. More than 2.1 million people are now living with HIV in Latin America and the Caribbean including the estimated 2,30,000 that contracted HIV in the past year. At least 1,00,000 people died of AIDS in the same period, the highest regional death toll after sub-Saharan Africa and Asia.

All the main modes of transmission coexist in most countries, along with significant levels of risky behaviour such

Table 2.2: Regional HIV/AIDS statistics, end of 2005

Region	*Epidemic started*	*Adults & Children living with HIV/AIDS **	*Adult prevalence rate (per cent)*	*Adults & children infected with HIV/AIDS in 2005*
Sub Saharan Africa	Late '70's Early 80's	25.8	7.52	2.4
North Africa & Middle East	Late '80's	0.5	0.2	0.058
South & South East Asia	Late '80's	7.4	0.7	0.48
East Asia & Pacific	Late '80's	0.87	0.1	0.041
Latin America	Late '70's early 80's	1.8	0.6	0.066
Caribbean	Late '70's early 80's	0.3	1.6	0.024
Eastern Europe & Central Asia	Early '90's	1.6	0.9	0.062
Western Europe	Late '70's Early '80's	0.72	0.3	0.012
North America	Late '70's Early '80's	1.2	0.7	0.018
Global Total		**40.3**	**1.1**	**3.1**

Source: UNAIDS/WHO AIDS Epidemic Update, 2005 (* Millions).

as early sexual debut, unprotected sex with multiple partners and the use of unclean drug-injecting equipment.

The Global HIV/AIDS Epidemic:

- *The global HIV/AIDS epidemic has claimed over 20 million lives.*

- *40.3 million people are estimated to be living with HIV/AIDS Worldivide.*
- *AIDS is now the fourth leading cause of death worldwide and the number one cause of death in Africa.*

Impact of HIV/AIDS on Women, Children, and Young People

- *Women make up a growing percentage of adults living with HIV/AIDS around the world, rising from 41 per cent in 1997 to 50 per cent in 2003.*
- *In sub-Saharan Africa, women represent more than half of adults living with HIV/AIDS.*
- *Teens and young adults have been particularly affected by HIV/AIDS.*
- *Young people ages 15-24 account for 42 per cent of new HIV infections and represent almost a third of the global total* of *people living with HIV/AIDS.*
- *Women account for approximately 30 per cent of new HIV infections. (UNAIDS, 2005)*

One of the crucial factors about HIV/AIDS is that it is different from most other diseases and consequently requires a radically different and broader response, one, which goes beyond the health sector. The various factors, which make it different from other diseases, are:

- HIV occurs through specific risk behaviour that are within the realm of private life—i.e. extra marital sexual intercourse, which is intimate and private and not open to public debate.
- HIV selectively affects two groups—young adults and the very poor. 80 to 90 per cent of those affected are young adults at the prime of their productive and reproductive lives.
- HIV/AIDS retains a long period of invisibility, AIDS appearing many years later. However the danger is

that during this period most are unaware that they are infected and continue to spread the disease.

- The prognosis for HIV/AIDS is bleak. Currently there is no vaccine and no medical cure. Treatment options are very expensive. HIV/AIDS is essentially an incurable and fatal disease as at present.
- HIV/AIDS destabilises society because of the fear, blame, and stigma attached to it. It threatens basic human rights and invades the right to privacy and human dignity.
- The epidemic is less visible and visible consequences constitute an urgent and massive threat to development i.e. deteriorating child survival, reduced life expectancy, increasing number of orphans and loss of the most productive section of the population.

Educating people about HIV/AIDS and prevention is complicated as India has many major languages and hundreds of different dialects. So although some HIV/AIDS prevention and education can be done at the national level many of the efforts are best carried out at the state and local level.

HIV/AIDS AND INDIA'S RESPONSE

India has a population of one billion, around half of who are adults is the sexually active age group, with a large number below this age group. The first AIDS case in India was detected in 1986, and since then, HIV infection has been reported in all States and Union Territories.

The spread of HIV in India has been diverse, with much of India having a low rate of infection and the epidemic being most extreme in the Southern States of the Country and in the far northeast. 96 per cent of the total number of nationally reported AIDS cases were found 10 of the 28 States and 7 Union Territories, the worst and highest prevalence rates are found in Maharashtra and Gujarat in the west, Andhra Pradesh, Karnataka, Tamil Nadu, and Pondicherry in the south, and Manipur in the north-east. In the southern states, the infections are mostly due to heterosexual contact, while infections are mainly found amongst injecting drug users (IDU) in Manipur and Nagaland.

Table 2.3: Estimated Numbers of Adults and Children Living with HIV/AIDS, end of 2005

Adults	5,000,000
Women	1,900,000
Children	120,000
Total	**5,100,000**
Adult HIV prevalence estimate	0.9 per cent

Source: NACO, 2005

The Indian National AIDS Organisation (NACO) estimates that 5.134 million people were living with HIV in 2004. This represents a slight increase from the 2003 estimate, and a substantial increase from 4.58 million in 2002.

Table 2.4: AIDS Data on December, 2005

AIDS cases in India	*Cumulative AIDS Cases*
Males	77,457
Females	31,892
Total	**109,349**

The statistics for AIDS cases may be a poor guide to the severity of the epidemic, as in many situations a patient will die without HIV having been diagnosed, and the cause of death attributed to an opportunistic infection, such as tuberculosis or PCP.

India has had a sharp increase in the estimated number of HIV infections, from a few thousand in the early 1990s to around 5.1 million children and adults living with IV/ AIDS in 2003. With a population of over one billion, the HIV epidemics in India will have a major impact on the overall spread of HIV in Asia and the Pacific and indeed worldwide.

Table 2.5: Estimated Numbers According to Transmission Categories, 2005

Transmission Categories	*Number of cases*	*Per cent*
Sexual	93,964	85.93
Perinatal	3,957	3.62
Blood and blood products	1,202	2.01
Injecting drug users	2,661	2.43
Not known	6,566	6.00
Total	**109,349**	**100**

Source: NACO, 2005

Table 2.6: Estimated Numbers by Age and Sex Groups, 2005

Age group	*Male*	*Female*	*Total*
0-14	2,779	1,945	4,744
15-29	21,440	14,149	35,589
30-49	47,132	14,159	61,471
> 50	5,906	1,639	7,545
Total	**77,457**	**31,892**	**109,349**

Source: NACO, 2005.

It would be easy to underestimate the challenge of HIV/AIDS in a large population and population density, low literacy levels and consequently low levels of awareness, and HIV/AIDS is one of challenging public health problems ever faced by the country. *"How do you talk to about HIV/AIDS to someone who does not know the basics about health and hygiene?"* Ratna Gaekwad, an outreach coordinator with the Delhi NGO Prayatna said.

The number of HIV infections in India is difficult to determine and the subject of ongoing controversy. India's prevalence estimates are based solely on sentinel surveillance conducted at public sites. The country has no national information system to collect HIV testing information from the private sector, which provides 80 per cent of health care in the country.

Although the HIV prevalence rate is low (0.9 per cent), the overall number of people with HIV infection is high according to estimates by UNAIDS. The official Indian figures do not reveal such a scale of infection, but weaknesses in the surveillance system, bias in targeting groups for testing, and the lack of availability of testing services in several parts of the country suggest a significant element of under reporting. Given India's large population, with most of the Indian states having a population greater than a majority of the countries in Africa, a mere 0.1 per cent increase in the prevalence rate would increase the number of adults living with HIV/AIDS by over half a million people.

A National AIDS Control Programme was launched in 1987 with the programme activities covering surveillance, screening blood and blood products and health education. In 1992 the National AIDS Control Organisation (NACO) was established. NACO carries out India's National AIDS Programme, which includes the formulation of policy, prevention and control programmes. The same year that NACO was established, the Government launched a Strategic Plan for HIV/AIDS prevention under the National AIDS Control Project. The Project established the administrative and technical basis for programme management and also set up State AIDS bodies in 25 states and 7 union territories. The Project was able to make a number of important improvements in HIV prevention such as improving blood safety.

Globally India is second only to South Africa in terms of the overall number of people living with the disease.

- NACO estimated that there the number of Indians living with HIV increased by 500,000 in 2003 to 5.1 million. Around 38 per cent of these people were women.
- In November 2004, NACO published the number of AIDS cases reported. The total of AIDS cases in India was 87,596 of whom 24,504 were women. This data also indicated that 37 per cent of reported AIDS cases were diagnosed among people under 30.

- The UN Population Division projects that India's adult HIV prevalence will peak at 1.9 per cent in 2019. The UN estimates that there were 2.7 million AIDS deaths in India between 1980 and 2000. During 2000-15, the UN projects 12.3 million AIDS deaths and 49.5 million deaths during 2015-50.
- A 2002 report by the CIA's National Intelligence Council predicted 20 million to 25 million AIDS cases in India by 2010, more than any other country in the world.

With the second phase of the National AIDS Control Programme (1999-2004), NACO has expanded its programme. NACO provides funds to State AIDS Control Societies for targeted interventions, blood safety, youth campaigns, Voluntary Testing Centres (VTC), care and support and social mobilisation. The second phase of the programme aims to promote cooperation among public, private and voluntary sectors. NACO sponsored prevention efforts have included concerts, TV spots with a popular Indian film-star, radio drama, radio programme and organising a voluntary blood donation day. School AIDS education programme in India include training teachers and peer educator among students, role-playing, debates and discussions. The programme has worked towards student youth to raise awareness levels, help young people to resist peer pressure and develop a safe and responsible life-style. (NACO, 2004)

However it is still debatable as to whether there is sufficient commitment to combating the epidemic at government level. Many Indians in positions of power refuse to accept that their country faces a grave threat from the epidemic. And as the epidemic spreads, the battle against AIDS is mired by a lack of consensus on the extent of the pandemic, the "right strategy" to combat it, and how to deal frankly with sexuality. But according to Peter Piot of UNAIDS: *"In order to prevent the spread of HIV, a combination approach is required. We need to promote awareness education, abstinence, delay of sex, faithfulness and the use of condoms. No single approach will work. "*

The Indian government is also criticised for clinging to the idea that the epidemic is limited to "high risk groups", such as sex workers, drug users and truck drivers, and that targeting them is the best strategy to contain the epidemic further. But this approach no longer reflects the reality of at least some Indian states, where the epidemic is in the general population. In these states women who only have sex with their husbands may be the group at highest risk of HIV transmission, and although in Indian society men can experiment with sex outside of marriage, women do not have the status to demand condom use of their husbands. There needs to be political leadership, and there needs to be effective action taken in respect of all aspects of the epidemic. *"At recent meetings in India, I heard great speeches, but as for action, zero.* " (Piot, Director UNAIDS, 2004)

The HIV/AIDS situation in different states: There are a number of states where the HIV prevalence in antenatal women is l per cent or more, and these are considered to be high prevalence states. The prevalence rates are from data collected during screening of women attending antenatal clinics (ANC), meaning that these prevalence rates are only relevant to sexually active women. However, these rates can provide a reasonable estimate of HIV prevalence within the general population in each state.

(a) Andhra Pradesh: Andhra Pradesh has one of the fastest increasing HIV/AIDS prevalence rates in India. In 2002 the ANC prevalence rate was 1.25 per cent and NACO has estimated that more than 400,000 people are living with HIV in Andhra Pradesh, the second highest number after Maharashtra State. This is 10 per cent of the total HIV cases in India and ninety per cent of the infections in the state occur through sexual transmission. Andhra Pradesh is a Hindu state in the southeast of the country with a total population of 75.7 million.

(b) Goa: Goa is in the southwest of India and is best known as a tourist destination. And tourism is so prominent that the number of tourists almost equals the population of the state, which is 1.34 million. HIV infections have increased noticeably in Goa in the past couple of years. The ANC prevalence rate increased from 0.5 per cent in 2001 to 1.38 per cent in 2002.

(c) ***Karnataka:*** In Karnataka the mean prevalence among ANCs was 1.13 in 2001 and 1.75 per cent in 2002. In 2001 there were four districts with an ANC prevalence of 2 per cent or more, and these are located in the southern part of the state, in and around Bangalore, on the border with Tamil Nadu, or in northern Karnataka's "devadasi belt." Devadasi women are a group of women, who historically, have been dedicated to the service of gods. These days, this has evolved into sanctioned prostitution—as a result many women from this part of the country are supplied to the sex trade in big cities such as Mumbai. Karnataka has a population of 52.7 million and is a diverse state in the southwest of India.

(d) ***Maharashtra and Mumbai:*** Mumbai (Bombay) is the capital city of Maharastra State and is the second most populated city in India with a population of 16.4 million people. Maharastra is a very large state and it has a total population of 96.8 million. The 2002 ANC prevalence rate for the state of Maharastra was 1.25 per cent and the prevalence for the city of Mumbai 0.75 per cent.

(e) ***Manipur:*** Manipur, a small state of 2.4 million people in the north east of India, has the highest concentration of HIV/AIDS infection in India. The ANC prevalence in Manipur in 2002 was 1.12 per cent and among injecting drug users at three surveillance sites the HIV prevalence was an extremely high 39.06 per cent.

(f) ***Mizoram:*** In 1998, in the small north eastern state of Mizoram which has a population of less than a million, the epidemic took off quickly among male injecting drug users; with some drug clinics registering HIV rates of more than 70 per cent among their patients. In 2002, the ANC prevalence was 1.50 per cent.

(g) ***Nagaland:*** Another small northeastern state, with a population of two million and where injecting drug use has again been the driving force behind the HIV epidemic. In 2002, the ANC prevalence was 1.25 per cent and the HIV prevalence among injecting drug users was 10.28 per cent.

(h) ***Tamil Nadu:*** When surveillance systems in the southern Indian state of Tamil Nadu, home to some 60 million people, showed that HIV infection rates among pregnant women were rising, tripling to 1.25 per cent between 1995 and 1997, the State Government acted decisively. It set up an AIDS society, which worked closely with non-governmental organisations (NGOs) and other partners to develop an active AIDS prevention campaign. The ANC prevalence in Tamil Nadu was 0.88 per cent in 2002, although an infection rate of 33.8 per cent was recorded at the one surveillance site for injecting drug users. By September 2003 Tamil Nadu had reported 24,667 cases of AIDS, the highest number reported to NACO by any state.

Although HIV/AIDS is still largely concentrated in at-risk populations, including commercial sex workers, injecting drug users, and truck drivers, the surveillance data suggests that the epidemic is moving beyond these groups in some regions and into the general population. It is also moving from urban to rural districts.

"In some parts of India, particularly the states that are reporting the higher prevalence, the tipping point is long past. I think there is absolutely no doubt that the virus is moving into the general population, " says Dr. R. Feachem, executive director of the Global Fund to Fight AIDS,

Tuberculosis and Malaria. In July 2003, Dr. Meenakshi Datta Ghosh, project director for NACO, stated that "HIV/AIDS *no longer affects only high-risk groups or urban populations, but is gradually spreading into rural areas and the general population.* "

The epidemic continues to shift towards women and young people. It has been estimated that 38 per cent of adults living with HIV/AIDS in India as of the end of 2003 were women. In 2004, it was estimated that 22 per cent of HIV cases in India were housewives with a single partner. The increasing HIV prevalence among women can consequently be seen in the increase of mother to child transmission of HIV and paediatric HIV cases.

The majority of the reported AIDS cases have occurred in the sexually active and economically productive 15 to 44 age group. The predominant mode of HIV transmission is through heterosexual contact, the second most common mode being injecting drug use. Previously blood transfusion and blood product transfusions were also major causes, but blood safety measures are now in place to prevent such transmission.

The Government responded soon after the first reported case in 1986 with interventions on surveillance, blood safety and dissemination, education and communication. In the initial years of the epidemic, AIDS prevention efforts were confined to 'hot spots' like Maharashtra, Tamil Nadu, Manipur and select big cities. Since, 1992 the World Bank has been funding a country wide National AIDS Control Project. The first phase of this project (1992-1999), with an IDA credit of $ 84 million, focussed on strengthening blood banks, STD clinics, surveillance systems and increasing awareness. Targeted interventions among high-risk behaviour groups were implemented only in a few states; care support activities received little attention in the first phase (India Health Report, 2004).

With more information about the epidemic since the mid-1990s, and learning from the experience of the first phase, the second phase of the project was launched in 1999 with IDA credit of $ 191 million. It focuses on targeted interventions among high-risk behaviour groups. In terms of management, state level autonomous societies have been established in the easy and timely transfer of funds, and increasing decentralisation and ownership of the project by the respective states.

In addition to the World Bank, state level AIDS Control Projects are also being implemented by several bilateral donors such as USAID of the US government (Tamil Nadu, and Maharastra), DIFD of the UK Government (Andhra Pradesh, Gujarat, Kerala, and Orissa) and Candadian International Development Agency (CIDA) of the Canadian Government (Karnataka and Rajastan). For 1999-2005, the World Bank outlay is rupees 11,550 million, that of USAID rupees 1660 million, and of DFID rupees 1040 million. While the World Bank project implemented through NACO covers the whole range of prevention, care and capacity building, bilaterally funded projects focus on the prevention of sexual transmission of HIV. There is a good degree of coordination between the World Bank funded and bilaterally funded projects, and government sponsored programmes, (India Health Report, 2004).

Evidence from successful AIDS Control Projects around the world, including some from India, indicates that the intervention programmes by peer educators among high risk groups are the most effective in containing the rapid spread of HIV.

This approach, now central to prevention efforts in India, clearly shows the rationale behind the interventions among core transmitter groups such as Commercial Sex Workers (CSWs), rather than among a widely dispersed group like the male clients of CSWs. Lessons learnt from successful Indian projects such as the Sonagachi project of Kolkata have been utilised on other parts of India. The STD/HIV Intervention Project in Sonagachi, Kolkata is one of the best examples of targeted interventions among sex workers. The project, implemented by an NGO, organised CSWs into informal groups and empowered them with negotiating skills for promoting condom use with their clients. Condom use has increased from nil in 1992 to over 70 per cent in 1993-94, and these levels sustained thereafter. Venereal disease Research Laboratory slide test (VDRL) positively has also reduced from over 20 per cent in 1992 to 5 per cent in 1998. This has ensured that the HIV prevalence are among CSWs in Kolkota has remained at around 5 per cent. In contrast, HIV prevalence rates among the CSWs in Mumbai rose rapidly from below 5 per cent in the early 1990s to over 50 per cent by 2000, (NACO, 2002)

Following the Sonagachi model, one study among CSWs in Andhra Pradesh has shown that condom usage among CSWs has gone up to 73 per cent, their knowledge of STDs and AIDS has risen to 92 per cent and all of them know where they can access services in case of need.

Similarly interventions initiated with prison inmates in eleven prisons in Andhra Pradesh have shown significant results in bringing about behavioural change among primary stakeholders and their spouses and in identifying and curing infections such as Tuberculosis and Sexually Transmitted Diseases/Reproductive Tract Infections.

While raising awareness level is not enough to change behaviour, knowledge about modes of transmission and methods of prevention ensure the success of intervention programmes. Tamil Nadu has been the pioneer in implementing highly effective awareness campaigns since the early 1990s, resulting in almost universal knowledge levels.

With a population of over one billion people, India is poised to suffer the world's largest HIV/AIDS epidemic if adequate action is not taken immediately. India needs a vigorous and sustained action to prevent the devastating effects of a full-blown AIDS epidemic.

❖ National AIDS Control Organisation (NACO) estimates that India had 5.1 million people infected with HIV as of the end of 2003. This represents a 10.3 per cent increase in estimated infections.

- In India 85 per cent of people that have HIV/AIDS were infected by a partner of the opposite sex.
- There is no cure for HIV/AIDS and the number of new infections occurring annually in India has not decreased in the last decade. Last year alone there were 500,000 new HIV infections (NACO 2003).
- The virus has started to spread from high-risk groups to the general population and to move from urban to rural areas.
- Nine out of 10 HIV positive people in India are between 15 and 44, the most economically productive age group (NACO 2003).

In 1986, the Government of India established a National AIDS Control Programme under the Ministry of Health and Family Welfare. Programme activities covered are surveillance, screening of blood and blood products, and health education. In 1992, with the support of the World Bank, the Ministry established the National AIDS Control Organisation (NACO) to coordinate an enhanced programme of preventive activities. NACO provided national leadership and facilitated the development of State AIDS Societies in all states across India.

With the HIV prevalence doubling, on average, every one to two years in certain groups, the challenge to keep pace with this rapid increase is immense. India requires increased state's commitment, more effective and efficient partnerships between the public sector and NGOs, donors and the international health community, and increased HIV-related work in other sectors (such as in education, transportation and rural development).

The Government has announced the National AIDS Policy and The National Blood Policy after a series of consultations with various stakeholders (NGOs, donors, people living with HIV/AIDS, civil society, and other partners).

These policies provide the necessary framework for strengthening national and state level response.

- ❖ India's plan focuses first and foremost on prevention. Its operational objective is to contain HIV prevalence at 3 per cent in the states with a generalised epidemic, 2 per cent in those with a concentrated epidemic and 1 per cent in the rest of the country.
- ❖ Aims to increase awareness to 90 per cent among youth and other vulnerable parts of the population.
- ❖ The Health Ministry has announced that they plan to provide Anti Retroviral therapy (ARV) starting from April 2004 to HIV positive new parents, infected children under age 15 and patients coming in to government hospitals in high-risk states (India Health Report, 2004).

In India, the Joint UN Programme is an expanded Theme group. Besides the UN family, it includes the National AIDS Control Organisation (NACO), bilateral donor agencies and the Indian Network for Positive People (INP+). It works closely with government, NGOs, community networks and other stakeholders in generating a well-coordinated and enhanced response to HIV/AIDS. Each member of the Theme Group takes the lead in its own specific focus area.

India received technical assistance and funding from a variety of UN partners and bilateral donors. In 2003, India received additional funds from new donors, namely the Global Fund to Fight AIDS, Tuberculosis, and Malaria (approximately US $100 million for care and support programmes) and the Gates Foundation, which has committed US$100 million over 10 years to strengthen HIV prevention among mobile populations.

The Bill and Melinda Gates Foundation's Avahan programme (2004) has donated most of its resources to focussed interventions in the six states with high HIV prevalence as well as along national highways. It aims to reduce HIV transmission among high-risk groups, especially sex workers, their clients, and Injecting Drug Users (IDUs), and to slow the spread of the epidemic into the general population. Advocacy, public education, and capacity building supplement these interventions.

More than 600 NGOs are implementing various HIV/ AIDS prevention and care activities, in particular for high-risk groups, through activities funded by the Government and other donor partners. Nearly 90 per cent of HIV infections in India have been reported from the 15-49 age groups, the most productive segment of the society. HIV has an intense negative impact on the workforce, business, individual workers and their families, as well as the economy at a macro level. Though the macroeconomic impact of the epidemic in industrial sector has been relatively low compared to the situation in Sub-Saharan Africa, the structural determinants of HIV transmission such as high level of poverty, migration, illiteracy, ill health, gender inequality and urbanisation are widely prevalent across the country.

The National AIDS Prevention and Control Policy recognises the need to take care of workers' health and welfare, in the organised and unorganised sectors, and the need for developing a multi-pronged response to HIV/AIDS in workplace.

The business community has personal and organisational skills, as well as local influences to reinforce the government and private efforts in the areas where the businesses are located. Some of the businesses involved in Workplace Education are Tata, Godrej Industries, and Colgate.

While raising awareness level through Awareness Campaigns alone is not enough to change behaviour, knowledge about modes of transmission and methods of prevention ensure the success of intervention programmes. Tamil Nadu has been a pioneer in implementing highly effective awareness campaigns since the early 1990s, resulting in almost universal knowledge levels. Several States are now implementing similar AIDS awareness programmes.

The current low level of HIV prevalence in India has not yet led to any adverse macro-economic impact. However, in select pockets where HIV prevalence is very high, there is evidence of adverse effects on families and communities. Well-known examples are the Commercial Sex Workers of Mumbai, IUDs of Manipur, and the transport workers of Tamil Nadu. Since the epidemic will worsen before it eventually levels off, it would be advisable to plan for these situations. This inevitable cycle in a HIV/AIDS epidemic is well documented in Africa: infections, followed by morbidity, stigma, mother to child transmission, mortality and orphans. India would do well to learn from the African experience and prepare for the future.

Adherence to the initiates such as Evidence-based Approach, Stronger political approach, Involvement of the Private sector, HIV/AIDS Awareness and Education, Support services for those living with HIV/AIDS and Collaboration with other Sectors—all government departments, NGOs, business, industry, community leaders and all the people can ensure alleviate the devastating social and economic impact of the pandemic (India Health Report, 2004).

HIV/AIDS AND ANDHRA PRADESH STATE'S RESPONSE

With 75.73 million population as of the 2001 Census, Andhra Pradesh is India's fifth most populous state in the country. It is also one of the country's six high HIV/AIDS prevalence states. The other states are Maharashtra, Karnataka, Tamil Nadu, Manipur and Nagaland.

Based on the sentinel Surveillance data, it is estimated by NACO (2004) that over 51,53,221 are infected with HIV in India an almost one tenth i.e. 5,00,000 above infections are in Andhra Pradesh. When HIV prevalence among high-risk groups (commercial sex workers, patients with STDs, men who have sex with men,) is five or more and one per cent or more among the low risk (women in antenatal clinics), a state is considered high prevalence, (NACO 2004).

Under the National AIDS Control Programme (NACP II) it was decided to address some of the identified issues on priority basis. Two broad problem categories are Prevention of HIV infection in High-risk population and prevention of HIV infection in general population. The interventions are designed to encourage safe sex behaviour among groups that are at greater risk of HIV such as Sex Workers, Truckers, Men having sex with men, Migrant Workers in Slums and Prisoners. Programme features include Behaviour Change Communication, STD Care and counselling, Condom Promotion and creating enabling environment. The targeted intervention programme implemented by NGO was increased from 24 in 1999 to 110 in 2004.

(a) STI Care

It is well established that presence of STIs increase the risk of HIV transmission, therefore encouraging the people to seek STI care is important. So far 85 STD Clinics have been strengthened to provide STD treatment apart from 140 CHCs (community health centres) and 1490 PHCs (primary health centres) under regular system.

(b) Condom Promotion

As a part of aggressive condom promotion mandate of free distribution and through social marketing, in A.P it was ensured supply and availability of condoms to right people at right time in right place. The approaches to link the social marketing organisation to the NGOs implementing their crucial role in the distribution of condoms to the needy.

(c) Information Education and Communication (IEC) Programmes

Several innovative programmes have been implemented to create awareness among general public as well as high-risk population. Innovative measures like partnering with barbers to create awareness on HIV/AIDS were started in January 2005, in addition to conducting seminars for policy makers, cultural troupes and work place awareness sessions. Legislative forum on HIV/AIDS was constituted and a Workshop for sensitising all the legislative members was organised in November 2004. All the 16 members of the committee are equipped with information on HIV/AIDS to conduct similar sensitisation workshop at Assembly constitution level. A workshop on sensitisation of religious leaders on HIV/AIDS was organised in December 2004 involving heads of all religious, with the objective of partnering with Faith based organisations on HIV/AIDS issues.

(d) Blood Safety

180 licenced Blood Banks are functioning in the state. Voluntary Blood donation is promoted through active involvement of Indian Red Cross, NSS and other voluntary organisations. As a result, HIV infection through blood transfusion has come down from 4 per cent to 1 per cent in the state.

(e) Voluntary Counselling and Testing Centers

Given the importance of voluntary counselling and testing for HIV, there are now 105 counselling and testing centers at teaching, district area hospitals and few CHCs. One counsellor is normally posted at each of the centers for providing quality service.

(f) Prevention of Parent to Child Transmission Centres

Testing pregnant women who might be at risk of HIV is a critical component of HIV prevention programme. Upon their consent women are tested for infection, Nevirapine tablet is given to the HIV positive mother during labour and delivery and to the child, soon after birth. The numbers of PPTCT centres have been increased to 41 by 2004 from 14 in 2002.

(g) School AIDS Education Programme

AIDS Prevention Education Programme (APEP) was taken up for 9th and 10th class students in schools 2002. This programme is encouraging students to adopt positive life styles required for prevention of HIV/AIDS. HIV/AIDS chapter is incorporated in 10th class syllabus.

(h) Colleges Talk AIDS Programme

"Colleges Talk AIDS" Programme was taken up for prevention of HIV/AIDS among the students of 5000 colleges in the state. It is proposed to launch "STOP AIDS" (Sustained Training and Orientation for Prevention of HIV/AIDS) programme in all the colleges through college students. This is meant for promotion of healthy life style among the college students.

(i) HIV/AIDS Awareness for Women

Capacity building of 30 lakhs women self-help groups was done in collaboration with Rural Development Department and Women Development and Child Welfare Department for prevention of HIV/AIDS in A.P.

(j) HIV/AIDS Awareness for Adolescent Girls

In collaboration with Women Development and Child Welfare Department 17,000 Anganwadi Workers were trained as resource person at Village and 9,28,000 adolescent girls were trained on prevention of HIV/AIDS.

(k) Youth Programmes

Under Awareness training programme on HIV/AIDS 2.10 lakh youth groups were covered. It is proposed to cover Youth groups in rural areas through Rajiv Yuva Sakthi groups.

(l) Capacity Building of Police Personnel

Training of Police personnel has been initiated in collaboration with A.P. Police Academy. Under this initiative around 80,000 police personnel would be covered for capacity building on HIV/AIDS.

(m) Work place Intervention

Awareness training on HIV/AIDS to cover 5 lakhs industrial workers is taken up through workplace interventions being implemented in collaboration with industries.

(n) Training of Medical and Para-medical Personnel

Capacity building and sensitisation of medical and para-medical personnel in both Government and private sectors including the non-qualified health service providers is going on. Capacity building at different levels is being done to strengthen the different components of service delivery such as STD care and Care and Support for doctors, nurses and para-medical staff.

(o) Care and Support

20 Care and Support Centers are functioning to provide services to the HIV Positive persons. 4 Drop-in centers are also working to provide services to People Living with HIV/AIDS. Drop in Centers are run by People Living with HIV/AIDS networks. Counselling services, treatment for opportunistic infection and referral services are provided in the Care and Support centers.

(p) People Living With HIV/AIDS Networks

The mobilisation of PLWHA (People Living with HIV/AIDS) networks is intensified through creation of positive people networks in all the districts in the state. These networks are helpful to address the psychological needs of infected. The PLWHA networks are also strengthened to play a very important role in expanding the prevention, treatment and care programmes for control of HIV/AIDS.

(q) Anti-Retroviral Drugs

Three ARV (Anti-Retroviral) Centres have been established in Osmania General Hospital, Hyderabad, King George Hospital, Vizag and Government General Hospital, Guntur for providing free ARV drugs to AIDS patients as per NACO orders.

HISTORICAL PERSPECTIVE OF HIV/AIDS RESEARCH

In the early years of the epidemic, preventing HIV was seen as an issue of changing the behaviour of individuals, particularly in high-risk groups. Survey research was initiated to locate individual risk behaviours in knowledge, attitudes and practices (KAP) studies.

Plummer (1991) stated that poverty and gender are intertwined in relation to HIV/AIDS. It is poor women and men that are most susceptible to HIV infections. Seventy per cent of the world's poor are women. Women are more vulnerable to HIV/AIDS because they have less secure employment, lower income (if any), less access to health care and social security, less entitlement to assets and savings and little power to negotiate sex. But poverty and socio-cultural norms and values are not the only reasons why women are more at risk of HIV infections, there are also biological reasons.

Bosompra (1992) reported on the focus group findings from Ghana on the Potential of drama and songs as channels for AIDS education in Africa. Education intervention by the Health Education Division of the Ministry of Health was imparted through a play entitled the "Bitter side of AIDS" which was performed in communities, churches and factories. Songs with AIDS related themes were incorporated in the dramas. After one month Questionnaire assessed awareness and knowledge of AIDS, impact of play and songs. The findings suggested that self-reported knowledge and behaviour change increased and that even after one month key themes of the play were remembered.

Kasule (1997) reported that in some villages in northern Senegal there is epidemiological relationship between migration and HIV status. His study found that 27 per cent of male work-migrants and 11 per cent their spouses were infected with HIV. In a control group of men and their wives who had not travelled outside Senegal in the last 10 years, only one man and one woman was infected with HIV.

The Global Programme on AIDS of the World Health Organisation (1993) reviewed 19 studies to examine the age of first sexual intercourse and reported levels of sexual activity among students who had been exposed to sex education. It found the following:

- There was no evidence that sex education leads to earlier or increased sexual activity in young people.
- Six studies showed that sex education either delayed the onset of sexual activity or reduced the overall frequency.
- Two studies showed that access to counselling and contraceptive services did not encourage earlier or increased sexual activity.
- Ten studies showed that sex education increased the adoption of safer practices by sexually active youth.
- School programmes that promoted both the postponement of sexual activity and the use of condoms when sex occurs were more effective in reducing risk than those that promoted abstinence alone.
- Sex education for youth is more effective when it is administered before young people become sexually active, and when skills and social norms (rather than knowledge) are emphasised. (WHO 1993).

Schopper et al (1995) reported the results of village based AIDS prevention in a rural district in Uganda. 30 community educators were recruited from every parish in the district and trained to conduct information sessions at the village level. Their educational work was supported by an illustrated AIDS information leaflet whose content was based on findings from a KAP study. A baseline KAP study was carried out on a cluster sample of (n=733) and women (n=753) aged 15-49 years. After 18 months the impact of the programme was measured through second KAP survey. Knowledge about AIDS increased from 26 per cent 63 per cent in women and 57 to 91 per cent in men. ($p<0.0001$). Condom use increased from 27 to 48 per cent. The main problem in interpreting the information is the lack of any control and the impact achieved was also may be due to exposure of the community to other educational activities.

Singer and Weeks (1996) remarked that public health campaigns about AIDS have often been directed towards individuals or to specifically targeted risk-groups, such as prostitutes and truck drivers. A group of truck drivers might, apart from driving trucks, not have very much in common and can belong to quite different social, economic and cultural groups. Hence, giving the same health message to a risk group may not be an effective way to halt the spread of HIV.

Elkins et al (1996) evaluated the HIV/AIDS education initiatives among women in north-eastern Thai villages. The methodology consisted of distribution of HIV/AIDS leaflet with pictures and few words to convey key messages on the nature of AIDS, transmission and the use of condoms. Every household received a leaflet. KAP questionnaire was given to women in 6 villages before and after receiving the leaflet. A second group of six villages were given the leaflet and post test one year later, a third group of 6 villages served as controls and were given a post test but no leaflets. The questionnaire measured knowledge, HIV/AIDS efficacy and condom readiness. Even among villages that had received leaflets, the major source of information identified by the participants were television and radio (89 per cent). There was no clearly demonstrable impact of the leaflet on most outcome measure.

Kagimu et al (1998) conducted an evaluation of the effectiveness of AIDS health education interventions in a Muslim community in Uganda. During 2 years of prevention activities in local Muslim communities, 23 trainers trained over 3,000 religious leaders and their assistants as "family AIDS workers" who in turn educated their communities on AIDS during home visits and at religious gatherings. Baseline survey (n=1907) and follow-up survey two years later (n=1826) Survey data was supplemented with data from project records, 9 focus group studies and 25 key informant interviews. Impact achieved was a significant increase in correct knowledge of HIV transmission, methods of preventing HIV infection and the risk associated with unsafe sexual practices and unsterilised circumcision ($p<0.001$). This is good example of an evaluation of a large-scale programme working through a religious institution.

The Swedish Government adopted (1999) a strategic framework that should guide continued support to research on HIV/AIDS. The strategy document "Investing for future generations" (1999) describes the stance the Swedish Government has taken as part of international efforts to prevent and mitigate the impact of HIV/AIDS. The strategy focuses on activities and support that address both immediate and underlying causes of the HIV/AIDS epidemic as well as its immediate and long-term effects.

Four strategic goals are established:

- ❖ To enable people to protect themselves against HIV infection (HIV Prevention)
- ❖ To encourage greater political commitment to HIV prevention programmes (Political Commitment)
- ❖ To allow people infected and affected by HIV/AIDS to pursue their lives with quality and dignity (Care and Support)
- ❖ To develop coping strategies to alleviate long-term effects (Coping Strategies)

A number of studies have been carried out in East and Southern Africa to determine trends in sexual and reproductive health knowledge, attitudes, practices and behaviour among young people. These studies show major gaps in many young people's knowledge of sexuality and reproduction (Kasule et al, 1997). Major obstacles to improving young people's knowledge of sexual and reproductive health are social attitudes, particularly the prohibitive silence around sexuality and the censure of pre-marital sexual relations.

AIDS is often called a disease of poverty (Collins and Rau, 2000). Poverty causes work migration and urban drift, and it causes women to engage in risky sexual practices, just to name a few examples. Being separated from their families for long periods of time, these people often find new sexual partners, or form new families. Employment opportunities in towns and industrial areas are usually very limited and this leads to the creation of an urban class of very poor men and women whose way of life may involve many sexual partners. For women, this can be a survival strategy, and as long as there are no realistic alternatives in terms of other income generating activities, women will continue engaging in risky sexual activities.

Bhuiya et al (2000) evaluated the effects of an AIDS awareness campaign in knowledge about AIDS in a remote rural area in Bangladesh. The activities of the AIDS campaign included rallies at village level by school pupils and large community gatherings. Surveys were carried out of 300 males and 300 females from 30 out of the 50 villages using a before the campaign and one month afterwards. The questionnaire consisted of open-ended questions. There was no control. 39 per cent of the respondents in the post intervention survey reported having heard about AIDS compared to 19 per cent in the pre intervention survey. The improvement in knowledge was similar across all genders, age and religious groups.

Simooya and Sanjobon (2001) conducted an "In but Free"—an HIV/AIDS intervention in an African prison. The target group consisted of 1300 male and female inmates in a prison in Zambia. As a part of the intervention the inmates nominated 5 inmates from every 12 dormitories to receive 3 day training as peer educators. Educational activities included peer to peer HIV/AIDS education, promotion of hygiene and drama on HIV/AIDS. The need for intervention was highlighted by the results of a voluntary testing programme in which 75 per cent of 99 inmates tested were found to be HIV positive. This report provides a valuable information and useful discussion on an intervention which targets an important target group.

Babola et al (2001) studied the impact of a community mobilisation project on health related knowledge and practices in Cameroon. The activities of the intervention involved selecting and training of community immobilisers from urban and rural communities and providing to them education on family planning, STIs and general child health promoted by the project. The project was evaluated through a structured questionnaire. The findings revealed that there was significant increase in knowledge on contraception ($p<0.05$), perception about vulnerability to HIV/AIDS ($p<0.001$), persons reporting have ever used condoms ($p<0.01$) and use of health care services ($p<0.01$) the impact was greater for all of these variables among persons exposed to the programme than not exposed.

UNAIDS (1999) observed that major criticism of some early AIDS prevention initiatives was that they failed to give enough attention to women's economic and social subordination and the implications of this for their ability to negotiate where, when and how sex took place. McGrath et al. (1993) gives an example from Uganda, where they found that women were well aware of the risk reduction messages given by AIDS control programmes, but because these messages failed to provide them with realistic alternatives, they continued to be at risk.

YOUTH /ADOLESCENTS AND HIV/AIDS

According to UNICEF (2000) over 50 per cent of young people (aged 15-24) in more than a dozen countries have never heard of AIDS or harbour serious misconceptions about how HIV is transmitted. Providing women and young people with candid information about AIDS and life skills is a prerequisite in any AIDS response.

African American youth are disproportionately represented among adolescent cases of HIV infection. The number of adolescents infected is doubling every 14 months. The primary risk factor for contacting HIV among adolescents is unprotected sexual intercourse. With 60 per cent of 12th graders from national sample reporting having had sexual intercourse a fairly substantial proportion of adolescents are at potential risk for contracting HIV. Because school connectedness is linked to later onset of sexual intercourse, most likely the 60 per cent estimate among 12th graders represents a considerable underestimation of the actual rate of sexual intercourse among 17-year old youth who have dropped out of school. Although each emerging cohort adolescents have been given awareness of the need to have safe sexual practice, less than 50 per cent of adolescents only use condoms consistently (Jemmott and Fong, 1998).

Greater wealth and changing lifestyles have increased the exposure of youth to new technologies and global culture. This is creating tension between traditional and modern values. It has led to new health risks, such as drug abuse, HIV/AIDS, unwanted pregnancies and abortions. Youth make up a growing share of HIV/AIDS infections from 10 per cent in 1994 to about 40 per cent today. Young women are especially vulnerable to sex-related health risks because of their limited decision-making power and lack of comprehensive sex education. (World Development Report, 2007)

Youth is transitional phase from childhood to adulthood when young people, through a process of intense physiological, psychological, social and economic change, gradually come to be recognised—and to recognise themselves—as adults. Youth is an important stage of life building the human capital that allows young people to escape poverty and lead better and more fulfilling lives. Young people are growing up in a more global world. Greater mobility and rapid urbanisation flow people across the borders are closely associated with new health risks worldwide. As a result, sexual initiation and sexual experimentation in youth carries far greater risks than before with very high HIV-prevalence rates.

In many ways the risks facing young people today are greater and consequences potentially more deadly, than for previous generations. This is most obvious in the spread of HIV/AIDS, increasingly prevalent among young people. A central element to HIV prevention is AIDS Education to change youth behaviour and encourage adoption of healthy life style. (World Bank, 2005)

Risk behaviour during youth can deplete productive human capital many years into the future. In some developing countries today, close to half of all young men are smokers. Similarly, HIV develops into AIDS with a lag of up to 10 years, taking its toll on people in their prime working ages. In many developing countries, new HIV infections affect young people disproportionately. The costs of treating AIDS are high and the treatments often ineffective. The best way to avoid the future loss of youth is to modify tire health behaviour. First, give them the knowledge to help them make informed choices about their behaviour and skills to negotiate safe behaviour with peers and partners. Second, create an environment for the youth to practice healthful behaviour.

Individuals may not have good information about the risks they face today, even if they understand the risks over time. More than half of the young in many countries are sexually active, and data from surveys conducted between the late 1990s and 2004 show that the proportion who initiated sexual activity before the age of 15 is increasing. A significant proportion of youth in developing countries especially girls are sexually active. Imperfect knowledge about consequences can lead people to engage in unprotected sex. Even in countries where HIV prevalence is high, a large proportion of young people engage in unprotected sex. These people are at greater risk of HIV infection. Education, often called a "social vaccine" is considered by many to protect young people from engaging in risky behaviours.

More than 100 million STIs other than HIV occur every year around the world among people under 25. Many infections, however, go unnoticed, especially among women and girls, who may show no symptoms or signs so mild that they are unrecognisable. Providing STI education and training providers to treat STIs in adolescents increased the uptake of STI services among sexually experienced students a significantly reduced the incidence of STIs. (World Development Report, 2007)

Programmes addressing youth are of particular importance in preventing HIV/AIDS. In 2003 the Ministry of health in Brazil launched a AIDS education programme in schools of five municipalities. In 2004 the programme was extended to 205 municipalities responsible for almost half of all HIV/AIDS cases in Brazil. The programme was expected to reach all public schools and this particular initiative has been Brazil's successful strategy of curbing the fast spread of HIV/AIDS.

Fitzgerald and Stanton (1999) reported that a curriculum based programme 'My future is my choice' in Namibia for African and American youth. It included basic information about reproductive health, HIV/AIDS, substance abuse and violence as well as communication and decision making skills over 14 sessions. The intervention was randomly assigned to young people in grades 9 to 11 (15 to 18 years old) in 10 secondary schools. Participants displayed improved knowledge of HIV/AIDS, reproduction and the use of condoms relative to the control group.

Interventions to change behaviour such as Abstain, Be faithful, use Condoms (ABC) have been the mainstays of HIV prevention since the 1990s. Providing accurate and specific information is more effective than providing vague or general information. School based HIV/STI programmes were more likely to have an impact on behaviour than general reproductive health programmes. A school based Sex/HIV education programme in Kenya that provided young girls with information about higher prevalence of HIV among older men reduced intergenerational sex and significantly reduced pregnancies among girls.

Inculcating life skills in schools is the surest way to enhance the capabilities of young people. This goes beyond skills needed for further schooling and work. School based reproductive health education programmes can increase knowledge and the adaptation of safe sexual behaviour. A school based sex education intervention in Kenya providing young girls with specific information such as the prevalence of HIV infection reduced risk behaviour among them.

Many young people are themselves living with HIV/AIDS or are coping with the deaths of parents, friends and relatives.

They have a key role in raising awareness about HIV/AIDS and supporting others. Many members of the AIDS challenge youth club in Uganda have had direct and distressing experience of AIDS, having lost parents or close relatives. Members are aged 13-35 years old, and the group meets regularly to share experience and ideas, and learn about AIDS and support others. During training courses, counselling sessions and club meetings members have build up their confidence and self esteem. They are open and honest in their family situations, and able to support others in affected families. They talk very freely about relationships, friendships, sex and condom use. Young people said that they had difficulties in talking about sex with their parents, and recognised their own responsibility to start communication by discussing neutral subjects such as work or school. Above all young people wanted to live with hope, not anxiety and fear. (AIDS Action, 1994)

KNOWLEDGE, ATTITUDE AND PRACTICE OF WOMEN AND ADOLESCENT GIRLS ON HIV/AIDS

All over the world, AIDS is becoming a leading cause of death among women. In many societies, in many cultures, being a woman is a significant risk factor for HIV acquisition.

Koichiro Matsura, (2004) Director-General of UNESCO, for International Women's Day, 8 March 2004, called to focus on the unique contributions, problems and opportunities that women face all over the world. It is both a celebration of achievement and a reminder of how far we have to go. The United Nations system is highlighting the many issues surrounding women and AIDS, which is also the mobilising theme for the 2004-2005 World AIDS campaign. AIDS is damaging and threatening many advances in human development, including efforts to improve the status and well being of women everywhere.

All infections by HIV, whether of women or men, are a matter of equal concern. At the same time, the recent dramatic increase in the percentage of women among adults infected by HIV is especially worrying. In 1997, women constituted 41 per cent of all HIV-infected adults. Just four years later, this figure had risen to 49.8 per cent and in 2003 it reached the 50 per cent mark. This pattern of growing rates of infection is particularly alarming among young women living in sub-Saharan Africa, where 67 per cent of infected 15 to 24 years olds are women. Globally, of the estimated 14,000 new HIV infections a day in 2003, almost 50 per cent were women. And there is no indication that the trend is reversing.

According to UNAIDS (2004) prevention is the mainstay of the response to AIDS, but is seldom implemented at a scale that would turn the tide of the epidemic. Effective, inexpensive and relatively simple HIV prevention interventions do exist, but the pace of the epidemic is clearly outstripping most country efforts towards effective prevention programming. Globally, less than one-fifth of people who need it have any access to prevention services.

UNAIDS (2003) Progress report estimates from 70 countries responding to a 2003 coverage survey, the proportion of pregnant women covered by services to prevent mother-to-child HIV transmission ranges from 2 per cent in the Western Pacific, to 5 per cent in sub-Saharan Africa, and 34 per cent in the Americas. In sub-Saharan Africa, nearly 60 per cent of primary school students receive basic AIDS education, compared with 13 per cent in the Western Pacific region.

Ndlovu and Sihlangu (1992) reported the results of an AIDS Knowledge, Attitude, Behaviour and Practice survey of high school students, which revealed various sources of first information about AIDS as newspapers, television, radio and magazine. Authority figures like health workers, parents, teachers and church leaders did not emerge as significant sources for first information.

Similar observation was made by Jimmott et al (1994) who reported that 92 per cent of the adolescents had heard about AIDS, largely through the mass media (79-85 per cent), with parents and teachers contributing in less than 40 per cent. Most of them knew that promiscuity, blood transfusion and sharing of injection needles and syringes are major modes of transmission. The study revealed that while general awareness of AIDS was good, detailed knowledge was riddled with misconceptions and confusion. It was recommended that health personnel should disseminate accurate information with the support of parents, teachers and the youths themselves.

Peersman (1998) stated that young people face a higher risk of infection with HIV because of their behaviours and HIV prevention programmes have failed to address their unique concerns. The report proposed a comprehensive health education model for HIV prevention for bisexual adolescents. The present health education efforts should be augmented by broader self and group empowerment training that would develop self-esteem, social skills, support networks, and access to risk reduction materials. Mutatkar (1998) also emphasised health education needs. He reported in his study that there was a decline in moral values in Indian culture and 50 per cent of male of 500 sample had pre and extra marital sex. The researcher concluded that awareness needs to be created in women at various levels and alternative survival opportunities need to be offered to poor and disadvantaged women.

McKusick et al (1990) study reports one of the most significant factors influencing knowledge, attitudes and behaviour in relation to AIDS is acquaintance with someone who is known to be infected with HIV or with that person's family, friends, and fellow workers.

Bassett, Sherman and Allen (1994) Study reported that many young people in Africa have adequate knowledge of STDs and HIV/AIDS but that does not necessarily translate into behaviour change. Adolescents were generally knowledgeable about AIDS, they know how the disease was transmitted and that it was fatal, but they did not think that they were at risk of HIV. Risk perceptions were instead projected upon "outsiders"—such as bar girls, prostitutes, homosexuals and truck drivers.

In Kenya, the Centre for the Study of Adolescence (CSA, 1995) has done extensive research and advocacy work, in collaboration with Kenya Association for the Promotion of Adolescent Health to promote adolescent reproductive health. Youth friendly services for STDs have been established by the Family Planning Association of Kenya (FPAK) in Nairobi, Mombassa and Nakuru. In addition, the Ministry of Health has established two youth clinics at Siaya and Machakos, funded by Sida. Other initiatives have included sports clubs, such as the Mathare Youth Sports Association The Kenyan Society for people with AIDS, working mainly with anti-AIDS groups in schools; Teenage Mothers and Girl's Association of Kenya which promotes female empowerment.

In Zambia, UNICEF (1994) has piloted Youth Friendly Services in Lusaka since 1994. There has been training of peer educators in Lusaka, the Copperbelt and Southern provinces work with young people. HIV/AIDS by Christian Children's Fund, Planned Parenthood Association of Zambia and Family Life Movement Zambia in Kafue. Family Life Movement Zambia is also providing family life education for young people in Southern, the Copperbelt and Lusaka provinces. Nationally, Planned Parenthood Association of Zambia has run skills training for youth and Family Health Trust has created Anti-AIDS Clubs in many schools.

Peruga and Rivo (1992) conducted a study to explore differences in AIDS knowledge between black and white American women. Findings revealed that primarily racial differences in the level of knowledge of preventive measures were due to differences in educational attainment and not to race. However, lack of awareness of the difference between asymptomatic individuals infected with human immunodeficiency virus and persons with AIDS remained significantly higher for black than for white respondents. This lack of awareness may facilitate exposure of a larger proportion of black respondents to HIV infection.

Srivastava et al (1992) conducted a study on 182 teachers from a random selection of 15 schools in rural area of

Lucknow district of Northern India. The teachers were interviewed to assess their awareness and knowledge about AIDS using a pretested questionnaire. Observations revealed that only 79.7 per cent of the teachers had heard about AIDS, newspapers being the main source of information. Many believed AIDS to be mosquito-borne and less than 2 per cent knew that condom usage make sex safer. The findings revealed that there is a need to undertake intensive health education efforts as school teachers are an important source of health related information for rural populations.

Kumar et al (1995) also studied teachers' awareness and opinion about AIDS in East Delhi. Observations revealed that majority of them were aware of various aspects of HIV/ AIDS. The study stated that teachers had some misconceptions regarding transmission of the disease, which was similar to the findings observed by Srivastava et al (1992). Most of them opined that they could play an important role on educating the students as well as the community regarding AIDS/STDs.

Elkins (1994) carried out a survey of mothers attending child health clinics in Thailand to determine their knowledge and awareness of HIV and AIDS. They found that the knowledge and awareness of mothers of childbearing age was very inadequate regarding HIV and AIDS.

Maticka (1994) conducted interviews with high-risk women in Thailand and found that knowledge, attitude, beliefs and practices among these women were inadequate regarding HIV/AIDS. Fajans (1995) observed similar findings. He had conducted a study in Indonesia to investigate knowledge and risk behaviour among commercial sex workers, which revealed that commercial sex workers had low levels of knowledge concerning HIV and STD transmission and prevention. Birru (1997) observed similar findings among commercial sex workers. He conducted a study among commercial sex workers at Miraz in Maharastra State. Findings of his study revealed that commercial sex workers had inadequate knowledge on AIDS and they had negative attitude towards prevention and control of HIV/AIDS.

Bajaj (1993), Muniammal (1994), Daniel, U (1995), conducted studies among student nurses, traditional birth attendants and multi purpose heath workers in Delhi, Chennai and Rajasthan, respectively using paper pencil test and found that the health workers' knowledge level was not satisfactory and also they had misconceptions on the transmission of the disease.

Agarwal (1996) assessed the existing level of knowledge of high school children about AIDS in Delhi. The study reported that overall level of knowledge about AIDS was high, but some misconceptions in knowledge regarding transmission, prognosis and prevention were found. Books and media were the most common sources of information. The study recommended a comprehensive school AIDS education programme should be developed to clarify areas of misconception among high school students.

Maswanya et al (2000) conducted a study to assess knowledge and attitudes concerning HIV infection and individuals with AIDS among female students attending colleges in Nagasaki, Japan. The study reported that the students demonstrated a high level of knowledge concerning HIV/AIDS, but had considerable misconceptions and prejudices about people having HIV/AIDS. The study concluded that low literacy, increased population, economic constrains, migration, urbanisation, sex tourism, bride supplying, flourishing sex industry have led to HIV spread from high risk group to general population.

Petro-Nustus and Wasileh (2000) conducted a study on University students' knowledge of AIDS on a sample of 1013 at Zarqua, Jordan. The results indicated the presence of knowledge deficit problem in terms of what can or can't transmit HIV /AIDS, taking into consideration that 54 per cent of the students stated that they 'knew very little about AIDS' 14 per cent said they never heard about AIDS. The results also revealed the presence of certain misconceptions (myths) concerning the students' general knowledge of HIV/ AIDS.

Todankar and Sumati (2000) conducted a study among the unmarried adolescent girls (12-19 years of age) of Bhil tribes in Maharashtra. The main focus of the study was: (1) to understand the knowledge, awareness, attitude and behaviour of adolescent girls regarding puberty changes, sex, contraception, STDs and HIV/AIDS; (2) to study the existing prevalence of premarital sexual behaviour; and (3) to understand the reproductive sexual health problems and treatment seeking behaviour of these girls. Both qualitative and quantitative data were collected through focus group discussions, in-depth-interviews, case studies and structured questionnaire. The study observed that very few girls had information about AIDS and misconception was widespread regarding mode of transmission. Involvement of adolescent girls in premarital sex was also noticed.

Singh (2001) conducted a study to assess the Knowledge, Attitude and Practice of Universal Precautions among Nurses working in the hospitals. The findings revealed that Nurses had adequate knowledge and positive attitude on HIV/AIDS but they had poor universal precaution practices. Their professional exposures to HIV/AIDS patients, duration of professional experience and in-service education made no significant difference in them.

Dhasaradhan (2001) studied the Knowledge and attitude of Nurses towards HIV/AIDS patients in Chennai. A sample of 100 nurses answered a multiple choice questionnaire on etiology, clinical manifestations, mode of spread, laboratory tests, treatment, prevention, precautions and self-protection and counselling of patients with AIDS. The study shows that the knowledge and attitude of Nurses in relation to the care of AIDS patients was moderately adequate. But those who have had exposure to AIDS Education programme showed adequate level of Knowledge and positive attitude levels than others. There was also positive association between knowledge and attitude of Nurses towards HIV/AIDS.

Vati et al (2003) studied about AIDS awareness among Hospital Class IV employees. The one group post-test design was adopted to evaluate the post teaching knowledge about HIV/AIDS. 808 subjects attended the AIDS education programme. The findings show that the knowledge of class IV employees in the health care setting was highly satisfactory after attending the Education programme of 6 hours of teaching which included lectures, discussion, demonstrations and return demonstrations.

PREVENTION AND CONTROL OF HIV/AIDS AND THE ROLE OF THE FAMILY, SOCIETY, GOVERNMENT AND NON-GOVERNMENT ORGANISATIONS

Although the role of families in caring for its sick members is as old as humankind, only in recent years have researchers, health professionals, and family practitioners recognised the important role of the family in disease prevention and health promotion. WHIV infection is now becoming a long-term chronic illness affecting hundreds of thousands of families. (CDC, 1998)

Families are considered by many researchers to be the single most influential force in the lie of children and adolescents. HIV prevention family programmes have typically taken the form of education about HIV/AIDS and interventions aimed at developing parental competencies that can influence adolescents' behaviours. Increased attention has been given to examining how families serve to promote or encourage adolescents to adopt responsible behaviour that decreases high-risk behaviours. In contrast, parental monitoring of adolescent activities delays initiation of sexual behaviour. ((Pequegnat, 1997)

Research has overwhelmingly demonstrated the role that families play in healthy development. The Quality of parent-child relations is also an important predictor of sexual risk behaviours. Adolescents who report distance from their families are more likely to engage in sexual behaviours at a younger age. Positive family factors have also proven protective sexual risk behaviours. (Miller et al., 1998)

Given the important role that parents can play in promoting the sexual health of their adolescents, particularly as it relates to HIV prevention, several parent oriented interventions have been developed by members of the National Institute of Mental Health on Families and HIV/AIDS.

Krauss et al (2000) has developed a prevention programme for mothers and fathers to use with preadolescent children to help parents become experts in their children's eyes. In this way parents can teach and be a model for their children's knowledge, attitudes and behaviour about HIV/AIDS and safer practices. These efforts are aimed at fostering family involvement in the sexual health of adolescents, including delay of sexual intercourse, acquisition of information about HIV/AIDS. These sessions cover HIV knowledge and HIV safety skills, communication about sex, drugs, and recognition of risky situations and how to avoid them, negotiation skills to handle risky situations and sensitive and safe interactions with persons with HIV. The initial parent training is followed by a parent-child session in which each parent and child met alone with a facilitator, the parent chooses activities to perform with the child, and the child has an opportunity to ask any unanswered questions.

Coping with AIDS is exacerbated when more than one family member in a household, or even in the close extended family, is HIV infected, including children. PWAs and their families are subject to considerable distress associated with these demands and concerns.

Rapkin et al (2000) have developed an intervention to enhance AIDS affected families abilities to problem solve. The family health project teaches families problem solving skills. Problem solving is broken down into its component elements, and families are encouraged to follow these steps: (a) create a comfortable climate for problem solving, (b) identify the problem, (c) brainstorm, (d) weigh the consequences of various alternatives, (e) think through together the implementation of possible solutions, (f) set goals and (g) evaluate solution outcomes.

Mitrani et al (2000) have designed an intervention to improve the quality of social relations and supports of African

American seropositive women. This approach focussing on changing the quality of relationships, building family trust, increasing mutual support, and reducing blaming and personal attacks was successful in helping the seropositive women regain a valued role with their families.

HIV/AIDS is considered a priority health and developmental problem and a matter of much concern for families, society, Government and Non-government organisations. Each community, region and country is continuing to make its efforts to combat this unprecedented challenge to human society by implementing national strategic plans with the involvement of all sectors concerned and non-governmental organisations.

In the 2001 UN Declaration of Commitment on HIV/AIDS, countries around the world committed themselves to massively scaling-up prevention programmes. The Declaration's goal is to reduce HIV prevalence among young people (15-24 years old) by 25 per cent in the most affected countries, and to reduce the proportion of infants infected with HIV by 20 per cent, both by 2005.

WHO goals and Strategies for prevention and control of HIV/AIDS: The over all goal of WHO's prevention and control programme is to reduce the risk of HIV transmission, and to alleviate the personal and social impact of HIV/AIDS.

The objectives of the programmes are:

- To prevent HIV transmission by promoting healthy life styles and interventions for disease prevention through promotion of safer sex, prevention and treatment of STIs, prevention of MTCT, and prevention of HIV transmission through injecting drug use.

- To improve the quality of life of those living with HIV/AIDS through treatment and care, including voluntary counselling and testing (VCT) psycho-social support, treatment of HIV/AIDS related disease and where possible anti-retroviral drug therapy.

- To alleviate the impact of HIV/AIDS on individual household and local communities by adopting and enabling health sector policies and institutional environments as part of wider social and economic development policies.

The programme will have the following strategies and interventions, which are in line with the objectives.

- Prevention of sexual transmission of HIV by: promoting community-based interventions among population at risk.
- Treatment of Sexually Transmitted Infections (STIs) by: integrating STI treatment services into primary health care and involving private practitioners.
- Prevention of transmission of HIV through blood and blood products by: ensuring safe blood transfusion with emphasis on quality, prevention of HIV among injecting drug users by dissemination of information on prevention of HIV.
- Ensuring safe skin-piercing practices at health care settings by: adhering to infection control procedures including universal precautions to be observed by all health care workers at all levels and in all health care settings.
- Prevention of mother-to-child transmission (MTCT) of HIV is by: primary prevention of sexual transmission and providing antiretroviral drugs to infected pregnant women and their newborn babies. (WHO, SEAR, 2002)

The WHO South East Asia Region will assist member countries in the achievement of the Global targets to achieve internationally agreed global prevention goal to reduce by 2005 HIV prevalence among young men and women aged 15 to 24 years in the most affected counties by 25 per cent and by 25 per cent globally by 2010. By 2003, implement universal precautions in health care settings to prevent transmission of HIV infection.

By 2005 ensure that at least 90 per cent, and by 2010 at least 95 per cent of young people aged 15 to 24 years have access to the information, education—including peer education and youth specific HIV education—and services necessary to develop the life skills required to reduce their vulnerability to HIV infection. (HO, 2002)

Halewood and Kenny (2006) report the results of HIV prevention programme: *Staying Alive* using Information Communication Technologies (ICTs) in Katmandu, where one-quarter of young use internet. More widespread use of television and radio makes these ICTs the main components in widespread information campaigns to prevent the spread of HIV/AIDS. The 2002 global HIV prevention campaign *Staying alive* was broadcast on television stations that reached 800 million homes, as well as radio stations in 56 countries. Survey results form three cities suggest that people exposed to the campaign were more likely to talk to others about HV/AIDS and more likely to understand the importance of preventive methods and discussing HIV/AIDS with sexual partners and getting tested for HIV.

In 1998 the United Nations High commissioner for Human rights and the Joint United Nations programme on HIV/AIDS together issued the international Guidelines on HIV/AIDS and Human Rights. The guidelines provide a framework for supporting both human rights and public health, emphasising the synergy between the two and offer concrete measures for protecting human rights in order to deal effectively with HIV/AIDS. (Human Development Report, 2000)

NACO, Government of India (1994) conducted a targeted intervention project for Truck Drivers and helpers for prevention of STDs/HIV/AIDS at Beltola, Assam along the National Highway 37 from Jalukbari to Jorabat. Some of the activities included Information, Education and Communication (IEC) and setting up of STD Clinic emphasising Syndrome Case Management of STDs. STD Clinic at Beltola along National Highway 37 was set up which treated a large number of STD cases and provided

Counselling and Condoms to the target population. Primarily, the target audience were the truck drivers, their helpers and women who sell sex along the highways and also the secondary stakeholders which include dhaba owners, petrol pump owners, clearing agents, weighbridges, saloons, pharmacies, hotels, pan shops, coal agents, tyre shops, police and other transport related officials including All Assam Truck Drivers Union and All Assam Labours Union in the project.

The AIDS Prevention and Control Project (APAC—Tamil Nadu) has conducted five annual rounds of behaviour sentinel surveys to track changes in knowledge and behaviour of certain high risk groups (CSWs, transport workers, and factory workers). The survey indicates rapid behaviour change among CSWs and transport workers in terms of condom use. Condom use among CSWs had risen sharply from around 55 per cent in 1996 to nearly 90 per cent and among truckers to nearly 80 per cent by 1999.

HIV/AIDS EDUCATION PROGRAMMES/STRATEGIES AND METHODOLOGIES USED FOR HIV/AIDS EDUCATION

UNAIDS/WHO (2001) state that the aim of AIDS education is to reduce the risk of HIV transmission, now and in the future. It is important that the education given should form part of an integrated national AIDS prevention and control strategy designed for that purpose. Vigorous prevention efforts are needed to equip women and young people with the knowledge and services (such as HIV/AIDS information, condom promotion, life skills training) they need to protect themselves against the virus.

To formulate strategy and plan for implementation of prevention and control of HIV/AIDS in India, Ministry of Health and Family Welfare constituted a National AIDS Committee in the Year 1986. The committee was formed with a view to bring together various ministries, non-government organisations and private institutions for effective coordination in implementing prevention and control of HIV/AIDS programmes. Actual preventive activities like implementation of education and awareness programme, blood safety measures, control of hospital infection, condom promotion to prevent HIV/AIDS, strengthening of clinical services for both STD and HIV/AIDS gained momentum from 1992.

Dutta (1993) conducted a study on 105 in-service nursing personnel who completed a two-day's orientation-training programme on AIDS. The same written questionnaire assessed the subjects of their knowledge relating to AIDS before and after the orientation training. The study reported significant improvement in percentage of subjects (from 7.6 per cent pre training to 51.4 per cent post training) with desirable level of awareness and knowledge by the use of this planned orientation training programme. The study stressed the importance of continuing education for nursing personnel.

Bajaj (1993) conducted a study to evaluate the effectiveness of the Self-Instructional Module (SIM) on AIDS for student nurses in Delhi. Based on the learning needs of student nurses the SIM was developed and validated. Researcher observed that SIM was an effective teaching strategy and that it increased the knowledge of student nurses on AIDS and its control and prevention.

Kuhn et al (1994) developed and evaluated an AIDS education programme in a high school in South Africa. The programme, which addressed the whole school community, aimed to raise awareness about AIDS using variety of educational methods and operating through a number of channels. Students knowledge of and attitudes towards AIDS prevention were investigated before and after the AIDS programme and compared to a neighbouring school, in which no AIDS education was conducted. The programme greatly improved student knowledge of HIV transmission and prevention.

Muniammal (1994) conducted a study to evaluate the effectiveness of a Planned Teaching Programme (PTP) based on the learning needs of traditional birth attendants regarding prevention and control of AIDS in Tamil Nadu, India. The study was conducted in two phases. In phase one, descriptive survey design was used to collect data for identifying learning needs of TBAs. The major findings revealed that Traditional Birth Attendants had inadequate knowledge regarding AIDS. In phase two, a planned teaching programme was developed and evaluated. The findings revealed that the TBAs exposed to PTP had significantly higher knowledge scores than those not exposed to PTP. Hence, the PTP was found effective in enhancing the knowledge of TBAs regarding prevention and control of HIV/AIDS.

Handa (1994) studied the effectiveness of sex education programme among high school students in public schools of South Delhi. A sample of 180 students participated in the study. Based on the identified learning needs of the students a sex education programme was developed and validated. The programme was evaluated for its effectiveness in terms of knowledge gained by the students after the administration of the sex education programme. Researcher observed that there was significant increase in the knowledge gained by the sample.

Daniel (1995) carried out a study to develop and evaluate the effectiveness of a self-instructional module (SIM) on HIV/AIDS: prevention and control for multipurpose health workers based on the identified learning needs in Rajasthan. The findings reported revealed that the mean post-test knowledge scores of experimental group were significantly higher than the mean post-test knowledge scores of control group suggesting that the SIM was effective.

Ray et al (1995) studied the effectiveness of "One day AIDS Awareness Programme" on I.C.D.S functionaries West Bengal. Pre-training knowledge and post-training knowledge about AIDS and perception of risk for acquiring HIV/AIDS were assessed. The percentage increase in mean scores was found to be 66.55 per cent, 76.6 per cent, and 57.1 per cent in 3 districts of West Bengal respectively.

The UNAIDS and W.H.O (1995) prepared a strategy to boost global response on prevention and control of HIV/AIDS. W.H.O through its regional offices has initiated the new challenges for global development and response. These include: AIDS and Human rights, Woman and AIDS, sex education in school, HIV infection in prison, vaccine development, research for female controlled prevention method.

W.H.O, SEARO (1995) developed a guide through a regional consultation of HIV/AIDS communicators and review by national AIDS programme managers of the member countries of the region. The guide presents a framework for Information Education Communication within a prevention and control programme for HIV/AIDS. It describes the steps in HIV/AIDS IEC planning implementation and evaluation. It provides guidelines for national AIDS programme managers on how to set priorities and systematically plan and implement IEC activities as part of AIDS prevention and care programmes.

The W.H.O support for country responses are (HIV/AIDS An Update SEARO, WHO, 1996):

- ❖ Programme Management, advocacy and support
- ❖ Promoting appropriate HIV prevention strategy and interventions
- ❖ HIV/AIDS care as a part of primary Health care
- ❖ Laboratory diagnosis and HIV/AIDS and STD surveillance

The three-prolonged global strategy adopted by WHO to tackle the epidemic calls for urgent action, commitment and solidarity to:

- ❖ Prevent AIDS infection
- ❖ Reduce the personal and social impact of HIV infection and AIDS by providing care and social support for the HIV infected their families and community.

- Mobilise and unify national and international efforts against AIDS

Parker (1996) reported that focus of HIV/AIDS prevention efforts has increasingly shifted from models aimed at changes in individual risk behaviour to models aimed at community mobilisation. Earlier emphasis on information based educational campaigns has given way to intervention programmes aimed at enablement and empowerment in the face of the epidemic.

Dark (1996) reports a successful and cost effective plan implemented on the campus of a small, urban college located in the mid-Atlantic region of the United States. Peer education programmes use student peers to act as role models, to become sources of accurate information and to support fellow students in their struggle toward learning, both academically and in life experiences. This method could address the need for adequate health education, especially in the area of HIV/AIDS among high-risk populations.

Visser (1996) study has shown that female peer educators can talk about sex without the risk of being stigmatised as promiscuous. Equipped with communication skills, educational materials and a certificate that recognised their role, peer educators can be successful in facilitating group discussions about sex and educating their peers about their bodies.

Birru (1997) conducted a study to evaluate the effectiveness of a planned teaching programme (PTP) for commercial sex workers regarding prevention and control of HIV/AIDS in Miraz, Maharastra. Interview schedule was used to collect data before and after the administration of the PTP. Major finding of the study revealed that commercial sex workers had inadequate knowledge in all six learning areas and they had negative attitude towards prevention and control of HIV/AIDS. PTP increased the knowledge and attitude scores of commercial sex workers in experimental group.

Pietrow et al (1997) suggests that mass media help raise awareness and improve knowledge of the epidemic. It can make people understand that there is an alternative to the situation within which they find themselves. Mass media and social marketing can play an important role in modifying concepts of masculinity and femininity and their relation to sexuality and HIV risk. Furthermore, mass media makes HIV/AIDS visible and puts it on the public agenda, which is a prerequisite for breaking the silence surrounding it.

Majumbar and Roberts (1998) conducted descriptive study in which they identified the need to generate culturally sensitive educational programmes and to evaluate such programmes for their effectiveness. Culturally sensitive AIDS educational training was offered to culturally diverse women. The study concluded that educational training had a positive effect on participants' attitude and knowledge regarding AIDS; they felt comfortable discussing their concerns in their own language, and with their friends from the same community.

Robertson and Lenten (1998) conducted a study on senior high school students regarding HIV infection in Bangkok. A survey questionnaire was administered before and after the administration of slide lecture presentation on HIV/AIDS. Knowledge about HIV/AIDS and risk factors in the post-test was significantly increased ($P < 0.001$) from pre-test status. However, their attitudes to an HIV infected persons were not significantly changed in the post-test.

Johns Hopkins University (1998) reports that about the effectiveness of a radio programme in which young people are encouraged to call in and talk about their questions and concerns. It builds on experiences made in the field of programming that AIDS prevention and information can be conveyed to young people in entertaining ways that capture their attention. Combining education and entertainment (edutainment) has proven to be highly effective in motivating young people to seek information and services in order to change health related behaviours. It captures the audience attention, evokes strong emotional responses and provides role models for identification and for behaviour change.

"NACO-APS (1998) for the first time in North East India, a Telephone AIDS Hotline Counselling Services Project for HIV/AIDS has been initiated by APS and supported by National AIDS Control Organisation. NACO-APS AIDS Hotline with Toll Free Telephone number—"1097" being operated by AIDS Prevention Society in Guwahati City serves the need of the young people to access information related to HIV/AIDS. There is a general need felt by the population specially the youth for a centre with services which could provide counselling as well as provide correct and simple information regarding HIV/AIDS in a user friendly environment safeguarding the confidentiality of a client. This line has provided callers with information related to HIV/AIDS including counselling, STD Treatment facilities, HIV testing facilities, HIV/AIDS care and support services etc. Thousands of callers benefited from the services provided by four counsellors in the project.

UNAIDS (1999) suggests that peer education is a widely used component of HIV prevention programmes among many groups of people and in many geographical areas. There have been projects to train members of almost every conceivable group as peer educators: primary and secondary school students, truck drivers, sex workers, hair dressers, taxi drivers, sports team members, farm workers to name but a few. Responses to these projects are often positive. People appreciate and generally accept as credible the information they receive from colleagues and peers.

Chaturvedi et al (1999) carried out a multi-method promotional package for enhancing awareness and knowledge on STD and AIDS among ITI trainees in resettlement colony of Delhi, India; using pre and post-assessment of the subjects for comparison. The study demonstrated that exposure to intensive promotional intervention even for a brief period can significantly raise awareness and knowledge of young people even on sensitive topics like STD and AIDS.

Valente and Bharat (1999) states that "Finally, there must still be strong informational programmes pointing out the reduction in the risk of AIDS from changed sexual behaviour". More important than discussing semantics i.e. whether to call inputs "education" or "information", is to discuss what works in AIDS education. There is a wealth of evidence that educational campaigns can be effective and arrest or reverse HIV trends by encouraging people to change or avoid risky behaviour and lifestyles.

Matthews et al (1999) carried out a community intervention in South Africa to evaluate the effectiveness of a drama-in-education programme. Seven pairs of secondary schools were randomised to receive either written information about HIV/AIDS or the drama programme. Questionnaire surveys of knowledge, attitude and behaviour were compared before and 6 months after the interventions. Improvements in knowledge ($P=0.0002$) and attitudes ($P= <0.00001$) about HIV/AIDS were demonstrated in pupils at schools receiving the drama programme when compared to pupils at schools receiving written information alone.

Vaughan and Asher (2000) reported that entertainment education on family planning and HIV prevention in terms of knowledge gain, change in attitude and behaviour was an effective measure among married women in Ghana. Their post-test survey showed an increase in their awareness of HIV and contraceptives improve important attitudes about fidelity and family relations and adopt family planning methods.

SAKHI (2000) An Intervention Project among Sex Workers: "Project Sakhi" is one of the first peer based intervention projects for prevention of HIV/AIDS/STDs among the sex workers in the North East India which has been implemented by APS in Guwahati City in Assam. The project, supported by Assam State AIDS Control Society, was started in March 2000. Recognising the poor sexual health status of sex workers in Guwahati city, the gateway to North East India, and their low level of knowledge, present belief systems, practices in prevention and care of sexual health, it was observed that it contributed to a situation where STD/

HIV could spread rapidly fuelling the need to have such an intervention project be implemented in the city.

Initially a baseline assessment was conducted through a sample survey to look into the issues of social demography, mapping, and behavioural practices among sex workers, knowledge and attitude towards STD/AIDS and assessed the prevalence of STDs among them. It was found that there is widespread prevalence of STD and a poor level of knowledge of STD/AIDS among the sex workers. There is also a high volume of migration and being the gateway of the Northeast, a large number of people enter and exit through this busy capital city. A very large immigrant population is also residing in various pockets of the city. Some sex workers in the city are young women from the neighbouring states and also from the neighbouring countries who cross over the porous borders.

Trained outreach and peers have effectively conducted behaviour change communication sessions and educated the clients on various issues of HIV/AIDS. Support from the community was evident as with their support a field based health centre was established to cater to the health needs of the sex workers. The project undertook activities for meeting the needs of the sex workers and addressed the issues related to education, literacy, childcare, education of children of sex workers and provided them psycho-social support.

AIDS Prevention Society (2000) has been involved in "YOUTH and AIDS PROJECT"—AIDS Education in Schools Programme since 1994. 20 schools were covered under the programme and another 25 schools are being planned to be covered under the project. AIDS Prevention Society was involved by NACO and UNICEF in the regional planning phase for AIDS Education Programme in North East India and APS was responsible along with State AIDS Cell officials of Government of Assam for preparing the State Plan for AIDS Education in Schools in Assam. APS Chairman, presented the paper "Need for Intervention with School Students" at the third Regional Workshop on AIDS education in Schools organised by NACO, Government of India in Aizawl, Mizoram State in Collaboration with UNICEF, UNESCO, UNAIDS and UNFPA.

Oakley et al (2001) studied 73 reports of evaluations of sexual health interventions examining the effectiveness of these interventions in changing knowledge, attitudes, or behavioural outcomes were identified, of which 65 were separate outcome evaluations. Of these studies, 45 (69 percent) lacked random control groups, 44 (68 per cent) failed to present pre intervention and 38 (59 per cent) post intervention data, and 26 (40 per cent) omitted to discuss the relevance of loss of data caused by drop-outs. Only 12 (18 per cent) of the 65 outcome evaluations were judged to be methodologically sound. Academic reviewers were more likely than authors to judge studies as unclear because of design faults. Only two of the sound evaluations recorded interventions which were effective in showing an impact on young people's sexual behaviour.

APS (AIDS Prevention Society, 2001) intervention with Injecting Drug Users (IUDs), Other Drug Users and Their Sexual Partners in Guwahati, Assam, supported by NACO, was one of the first harm reduction projects for Injecting Drug Users in the country along with Manipur and Nagaland states of North East India. The intervention is based on the Outreach Model, the project through trained Peer Educators provided services with the principles of Harm Reduction for the Injecting Drug Users and those Drug Users at risk of injecting and sharing injecting equipment. The principal objective of the project is aimed at:

- Increasing awareness of HIV/AIDS transmission among the injecting drug users, other drug users at risk of injecting and their sexual partners in Guwahati City.
- Reducing the incidence of sharing of injecting equipment used for injecting drugs by a large number of injecting drug users of Guwahati City in Assam.
- Safer injecting and safer sexual practices—Clean needle and syringes, reducing sharing practices and increasing proper condom use.

The NACO's (2001) National Baseline Behavioural Surveillance Survey reports that 5.9 per cent of high-risk males in Kolkata city had never heard of AIDS, compared with 3.7 per cent high-risk males in Bangalore, 2.3 per cent in Delhi, 2.2 per cent in Chennai and 1.1 per cent in Mumbai. In addition, the study showed widespread misconceptions about how the virus is transmitted, with 30 per cent of the individuals surveyed in Kolkata saying that sharing a meal could spread HIV, compared with 11.5 per cent, 13.4 per cent and 15.7 per cent in Bangalore, Mumbai and Delhi, respectively, and 45.2 per cent of people surveyed in Kolkata saying that mosquitoes spread HIV. Approximately 89.7 per cent of individuals surveyed in Chennai, 88.5 per cent in Bangalore, 81.3 per cent in Delhi and 75.6 per cent in Mumbai correctly identified the spread of HIV by mosquitoes to be a "complete" misconception.

Kirby et al (2002) studied school-based programmes to reduce sexual risk behaviours with a view to review of effectiveness of Sex and AIDS education programmes in U.S Schools. The authors identified 23 school based programmes and measured programme impact on behaviour. They then summarised the results of those studies, identifying the distinguishing characteristics of effective programmes, and citing important research questions to be addressed in the future. Not all sex and AIDS education programmes had significant effects on adolescent sexual risk-taking behaviour, but specific programmes did delay the initiation of intercourse, reduce the frequency of intercourse, reduce the number of sexual partners, or increase the use of condoms or other contraceptives. These effective programmes have the potential to reduce exposure to unintended pregnancy and sexually transmitted disease, including HIV infection. Additional research is needed to improve the effectiveness of programmes and to clarify the most important characteristics of effective programmes.

Ghosh (2002) from Times of India reports that the survey by Times of India revealed that the ignorance about HIV in India is attributed to the relative lack of AIDS awareness programmes. Only 11.9 per cent of respondents in the Kolkata reported having attended an AIDS awareness programme, compared with 85.3 per cent in Chennai, 72.1 per cent in Mumbai, 54.8 per cent in Bangalore and 37.1 per cent in Delhi. The area has also seen an increase in new HIV infections, with West Bengal recording 1,131 new cases in 2002 — more than the total number of HIV cases recorded in the previous decade in the state.

AIDS Prevention Society (APS, 2002) has conducted regular awareness programmes in various parts Guwahati City in Assam using IEC materials. This generated a lot of interest among the general population at the street level and there was always a very interesting and busy question and answer session after each session in the street. The programmes are organised in busy places of the city like bus stations, railway stations, market places, autorickshaw stands, in front of cinema houses and other busy public places. The need to conduct awareness programmes at street level for the general public was because the AIDS messages through public hoarding and signboards did not mean much for the people on the street as many among them hardly get the message or do not understand these messages.

The Government India (2003) has announced the National AIDS Policy and The National Blood Policy after a series of consultations with various stakeholders (NGOs, donors, people living with HIV/AIDS, civil society, and other partners). These policies provide the necessary framework for strengthening national and state level response. India's plan focuses first and foremost on prevention. Its operational objective is to contain HIV prevalence at 3 per cent in the states with a generalised epidemic, 2 per cent in those with a concentrated epidemic and 1 per cent in the rest of the country. Aims to increase awareness to 90 per cent among youth and other vulnerable parts of the population. The Health Ministry has announced that they plan to provide anti-retroviral therapy (ARV) starting April 2004 to HIV positive new parents, infected children under age 15 and patients coming in to government hospitals in high-risk states.

Heffernan (2004) from National AIDS Control Organisation (NACO) survey reports that India had 5.1 million people infected with HIV as of the end of 2003. This represents a 10.3 per cent increase in estimated infections. In India 85 per cent of people that have HIV/AIDS were infected by a partner of the opposite sex. The survey reveals that the virus has started to spread from high-risk groups to the general population and to move from urban to rural areas. Nine out of 10 HIV positive people in India are between 15 and 44, the most economically productive age group. Indian women are more at risk in getting infected by the HIV virus due to discrimination, lack of education, social standing and poverty. Today 1.9 million women are HIV positive. It was estimated that 22 per cent of HIV cases in India were housewives with a single partner.

According to NACO (2004) the impact of HIV/AIDS on Children and Youth is that 300,000 children between the ages 0-14 are HIV positive and the majority of the newly infected people in India are under 25 years.

The Bill and Melinda Gates Foundation's Avahan programme (2004), has devoted most of its resources to focussed interventions in the six states with high HIV prevalence as well as along national highways. It aims to reduce HIV transmission among high-risk groups, especially sex workers, their clients, and injecting drug users (IDUs), and to slow the spread of the epidemic into the general population. Advocacy, public education, and capacity building supplement these interventions.

CHARCA (2005) is a joint UN programme aimed at young women and girls in India for prevention of and education about HIV and other sexually transmitted infections. According to UN experts, women account for about 40 per cent of HIV cases in India, and there has been a recent rise in HIV prevalence among women and girls ages 15 to 24. "India has the right laws, policies and money, but implementation is an issue which needs to be addressed."

UNAIDS Country Coordinator Denis Broun said at a news conference, adding, "The need of the hour is to reach out to young women living in extremely difficult and marginal circumstances". Broun said that in addition to a lack of awareness about the virus in Indian communities, women's "vulnerability" to HIV often is because of their husbands, with about 80 per cent of new HIV cases among women last year occurring within marriage. Archana Tamang, chief of the women's human rights said that women also are at greater risk of contracting HIV because of biological differences, gender disparities, lack of education and sex trafficking. More than two million HIV-positive girls and women live in India (New Indian express, 3rd March 2006).

The new campaign, titled "Commitment to Protect the Young and Vulnerable," aims to use rock concerts, plays and skits in the Indian cities of Aizawl, Udaipur and Bellary. "We look at it as an advocacy tool using the popular format of music to draw the attention of policymakers at both the national and state levels," Alankar Malviya—a project coordinator for CHARCA said, adding, "It is clear that by dedicating the International Women's Day (March 8, 2004) to the issue of reducing women's growing susceptibility to the disease, we recognise the enormity of it"

The New Indian Express (March 3rd 2006) reported that the Coordinated HIV/AIDS Response Through Capacity Building and Awareness along with the United Nations Development Fund for Women, UNAIDS and Indian Government Agencies began Awareness Campaign to increase HIV/AIDS awareness among young women and girls in India ages 15 to 29.

Hussein, from Hindustan Times, (March 2006) reports about HIV Positive Woman Is Running for Legislature in India's Assam State. An HIV positive woman who advocates for increased HIV/AIDS awareness and heads the Assam Network of Positive People submitted an application to run for an Assembly seat in the Indian State of Assam.

The general spread of education be it formal, non-formal or informal empowers women and men to improve their lives and reduce the risks they face. Women who are educated are better equipped to demand and obtain their rights, and therefore to remain free from HIV infection. In many of the hardest-hit countries, educated women have been at the forefront of community mobilisation against HIV/AIDS. Thus, achieving the goals of Education for All, notably the commitments that focus on gender equality in education, is a vital contribution to HIV prevention. Ultimately, empowerment through education contributes to building secure relationships based on gender equality, mutual respect and consent.

Several National and International health agencies have prepared educational and teaching materials for specific groups. A few are described below:

National AIDS Control Organisation (1995) developed a Self-Instructional and Teaching Module for pre-service and in-service nurses and midwives on HIV Infection/AIDS: Prevention and control. The content was presented in five modules: (i) Epidemiological and transmission of HIV infection; (ii) HIV infection and disease; (iii) HIV transmission in Health Care Settings; (iv) Psychological impact of HIV infection on the individual and the community; (v) Developing Counseling skills; (vi) Health education; (vii) Nursing care of the Adult with HIV disease; (viii) The impact of HIV infection and HIV-related illness on women; (ix) Nursing care of the infant and child with HIV infection.

National AIDS Control Organisation (NACO, 1995) has launched massively nationwide programme known as "Family Health Awareness Campaign" which has twin objectives: i) to impart accurate information on the causes, consequences and treatment of STDs and HIV and ii) facilitating accessibility to services through the existing primary care system in the country. The programme has generated tremendous enthusiasm in the community, particularly women in seeking information and reproductive tract infections and their treatment at primary health centers. HIV/AIDS related information has been integrated with this campaign.

World Health Organisation (1996) has developed a handbook on AIDS Home Care. The draft of this South East Asia Regional Office (SEARO) edition of the hand book was developed and reviewed by a team of experts from different countries in the region. The aims of AIDS home care are:

- To prevent problems when possible
- To take care of existing problems, and
- To know when it is time to get help

The AIDS home care deals extensively with HIV/AIDS prevention and control in a simple and understandable language and supported by illustrations and figures. The content is presented under the following headings: (1) teaching people with AIDS and their families; (2) from HIV infection to AIDS; 3) living positively with AIDS; (4) women, children and HIV; (5) care of the dying; (6) management of common AIDS symptoms in the home; (7) conditions that need special attention in people with AIDS; and 8) general guide on the use of medications.

Central Health Education Bureau (CHEB, 1998) has developed AIDS information for Health care workers for protection against AIDS. It has emphasised (1) facts about AIDS; (2) AIDS transmission; (3) the clinical material that can transmit HIV; 4) How HIV the virus causing AIDS can be inactivated; (5) How HIV infection and AIDS can be prevented; (6) collection of blood specimen; (7) transport of specimen, (8) safe house keeping; (9) laundry and linen care, (10) toilet and sluice care, (11) infective waste disposal; (12) care of dietary services, and (13) management and notification of parentral or Mucous membrane exposures. This information has been widely used in health care settings to prevent the transmission of HIV infection.

Times of India (1998) the English daily newspaper developed and published an education material titled "AIDS Concerns All" in collaboration with UNICEF and NCERT. The content of the material included AIDS: the challenges ahead, are we prepared to face it?

Understanding the pandemic, Prevention is cure, Blood safety, Children and AIDS, Youth and AIDS, Women and AIDS.

Voluntary Health Association of India (VHAI, 1998) developed a better care series booklet on HIV/AIDS for everybody to know about HIV/AIDS. It contains information under following headings: (1) What is AIDS? (2) Where does HIV live in the body? (3) How does HIV enter the body? (4) Why should I worry about AIDS, (5) Can I identify a person with HIV/AIDS? (6) You can get HIV/AIDS from, (7) what happens to a person infected with HIV? (8) What can I do to keep HIV away, (9) Safe sex by use of condom, and (10) Do not inject drugs and safe blood transfusion. It was reported by VHAI (1993) that this booklet was found highly effective in enhancing the knowledge of HIV/AIDS in general population.

National AIDS Control Organisation (NACO, 2000) also developed an education package titled "What is AIDS?" The important aspects of the content presented include; Definition, Causes, Process of infection, Symptoms, Diagnosis, How to avoid AIDS.

UNICEF, UNAIDS, WHO (2004) advocacy publication "Opportunity in Crisis" makes a compelling case for the need to focus on young people as a central component of national AIDS control programmes. It includes a range of statistics, including detailed tables of national and regional data that clearly show young people are at the centre of the epidemic, and explain why they are particularly vulnerable to HIV/AIDS. In addition, "Opportunity in Crisis" outlines a ten-step strategy for accelerated action to prevent HIV/AIDS among young people that includes fighting silence and stigma, increasing access to core interventions such as information, skills and services, decreasing young people's vulnerability and ensuring that they have opportunities to participate.

SUMMARY OF THE CHAPTER

This chapter dealt with the review of research and non-research literature on HIV/AIDS Concept and definition,

India and Andhra Pradesh State's response to HIV/AIDS. Literature was focused on knowledge, attitude and practice of women regarding HIV/AIDS, strategies, and methodologies used for education, for prevention and control of HIV/AIDS. The review included both descriptive and experimental studies. Most studies used questionnaire and interview schedule to elicit the information. Findings of majority of the studies reflected inadequate knowledge about HIV/AIDS both in India and in abroad.

The literature review helped to design the study, to develop tools, collection of data and data analysis. Literature revealed many programmes used on AIDS education. Only few studies have tested the effectiveness of such programmes on HIV/AIDS. So far, only a few studies were found in India on HIV/AIDS education for women and adolescent girls increasing their awareness to HIV/AIDS prevention and control.

3 Methodology

Research methodology, is a way of systematically solving the research problem. It explains, the steps that are generally adopted by a researcher in studying the research problem along with the logic behind it. Methodology of research indicates the general pattern of organising the procedure for gathering valid and reliable data of the problem under investigation. This chapter deals with the methodology adopted for the study. It includes the research approach, design for the study, the setting, sample and sampling technique, development of the tools, preparation of AIDS Education Programme, development of AIDS Education Manual in print and electronic multi media, pilot study, data collection procedure and plan of data analysis.

RESEARCH APPROACH

The present study is an action research, testing an educational intervention to develop a replicable education intervention programme for control of HIV/AIDS. In this study the primary aim of the researcher was to find the effectiveness of AIDS Education Programme (AEP), in terms of gain in knowledge, attitude and practice among adolescent girls from selected Junior colleges and to find association between the knowledge, attitude and practice and selected independent variables.

RESEARCH DESIGN

Polit and Hungler (1999) state that a research design incorporates the most important methodological decisions that the researcher makes in conducting a research study. It depicts the overall plan for organisation of scientific investigation.

The research design indicates various steps in the research project followed by the researcher. It served the investigator as blue print to execute the research project as planned.

The present study was an action research and the research design was based on *Systems model* (WHO SEARO Technical Publications No: 6, 1985). The model consists of *three phases: input, process, output* and a *context* (*See Figure 3.l on next page*). These three phases are interdependent and components of one phase are carried over to the next phase and vice versa.

Input: The Adolescent girls from Junior Colleges with their background and existing characteristics such as demographic profile, their exposure to mass media on HIV/AIDS and their existing knowledge, attitude and practice regarding HIV/AIDS were collected, in order to develop a need based educational programme which will constitute the input for the present study.

Process: The process included the development of the tools on demographic profile and exposure of the sample to mass media, development of scales on HIV/AIDS knowledge, attitude and practice and assessment of knowledge, attitude and practice on HIV/AIDS using these tools. Process also refers to the different operational procedures in the overall implementation of AIDS Education Programme (AEP). The different activities in the process include development of AIDS Education Programme, objectives, checklist for validation, preparation of messages for the AIDS Education Programme, development of AIDS Education Manual in print and electronic multi media and administration of AIDS Education Programme using the AIDS Education Programme Manual and electronic multi media to Junior college students.

Figure 3.1
Research Design

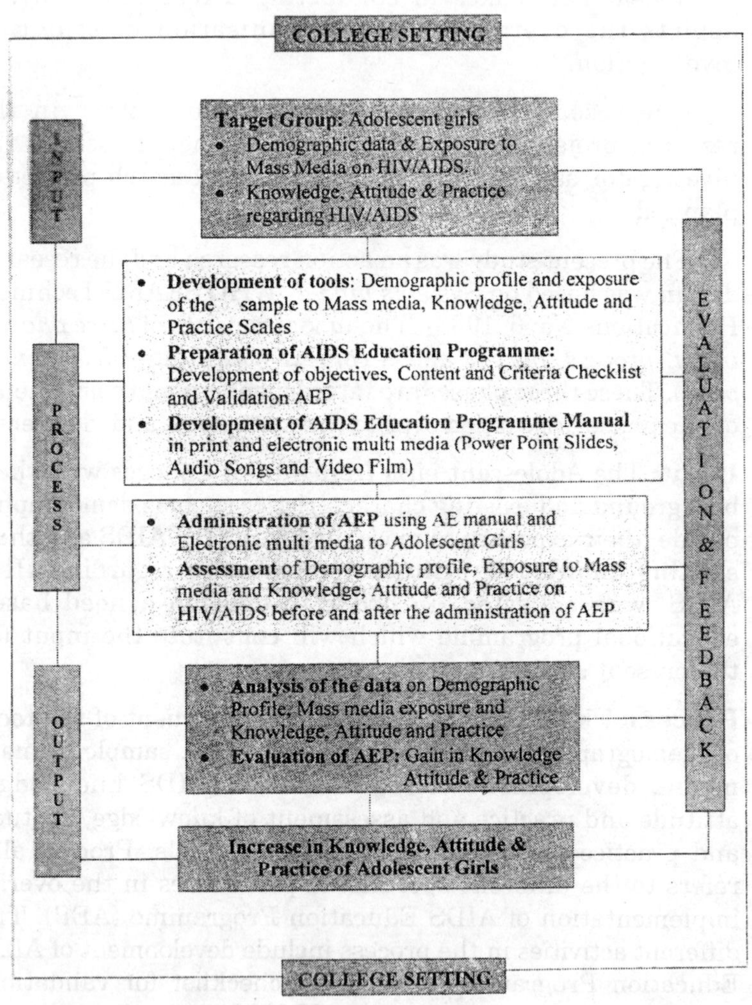

Output: The Output was evaluated by analysing the Demographic profile and exposure of the sample to mass media and the knowledge, attitude and practice gained by adolescent girls on HIV/AIDS after the administration of the AIDS Education Programme.

Context: Context refers to the environment in which the AIDS Education Programme took place. In the present study, the context referred to Junior Colleges for girls, where the target group was living at the time of the study.

The AIDS Education Programme designed for the present study consisted of experimental and control groups. The knowledge, attitude and practice of the sample was pre-tested, post-tested (1) and again post tested (II), which was a true experimental design to measure the effectiveness of AIDS Education Programme on a randomly selected 360 sample from two selected Junior Colleges for Girls. The AIDS Education Programme and study design of the present investigation in brief and details are presented in Table 3.1 and Table 3.2.

Table 3.1: AIDS Education Programme

Group	*Pre-test Intervention*	*Educational*	*Post-test I*	*Educational Intervention*	*Post-test II*
RE	TI	X1	T2	X2	T3
RC	T4	–	T5	–	–

KEY

RE : Randomised Experimental Group

RC : Randomised Control Group

T1, T4 : Knowledge, Attitude and Practice Pre-tests

T2, T5 : Knowledge, Attitude and Practice Post-test I

T3 : Knowledge, Attitude and Practice Post-test II

X1 : Educational Intervention—AIDS Education Programme

X2 : Peer Group Discussion/Reinforcement of AEP

The schematic representation of the present study describes the phases of the study as given in Table 3.2.

Table 3.2: Schematic Representation of the Study Design

Group	*Pre-test*	*Educational Intervention*	*Post-test I*	*Educational Intervention*	*Post-test II*
Day1	2, 3 & 4	30	150, 151	180	
Experimental 180 Junior College Girl Students	DP & KAP-Pre	A E P	KAP-Post I	RAEP/PGD	KAP-Post II
Control 180 Junior College Girl Students	DP & KAP-Pre	–	KAP-Post I	–	–

KEY

DP : Demographic Profile of the Sample

KAP-Pre : Knowledge, Attitude and Practice Pre-test

AEP : AIDS Education Programme

KAP-Post I : Knowledge, Attitude and Practice Post-test I

RAEP/PGD : Reinforcement AEP/Peer Group Discussion

KAP-Post II : Knowledge, Attitude and Practice Post-test II

The study design explains various steps in the research project followed by the researcher. In the first phase the researcher assessed data on demographic profile, exposure to mass media and knowledge, attitude and practice pre-test from the subjects. In the second phase the AIDS Education Programme was conducted for one hour daily using the AIDS Education Programme Manual and Electronic Multi-media for three days. In the third phase knowledge, attitude and practice post-test I was conducted after exactly a month (30 days). After a gap of 4 months i.e. on days 150 and 151, the same sample had an AIDS Education Programme again as a reinforcement followed by Peer group discussion on HIV/ AIDS. On day 180 post-test II was given using the same tools. This enabled the researcher to strongly motivate the subjects for consistent increase in their knowledge, develop positive attitude and favourable practice regarding HIV/AIDS.

LOCALE OF THE STUDY

Guntur District in Andhra Pradesh was selected as the study area. According to the Board of Intermediate Education, Hyderabad, there are 188 Junior Colleges in the District. About 35 Junior Colleges are managed by the Government, while 22 Junior colleges are managed by the private organisations but are aided by the Government. The rest of the Junior colleges are managed and supported by the private managements themselves. Out of these 188 Junior Colleges, 20 Junior colleges are for Girls. (*See Figure 3.2 on next page*)

SAMPLE SELECTION

The study was conducted at St. Joseph's Junior College for Girls (StJJC), Nallapadu, and St. Ann's Junior College for Girls (StAJC), Guntur District, Andhra Pradesh. St. Joseph's Junior college for Girls is 7 km from Guntur City, belonging to Guntur Municipality area. This college offers Intermediate courses to 750 Girl students, studying both Physical and Biological Sciences as well as Arts groups such as Civics, Economics, Commerce and History. St. Ann's Junior College for Girls is situated in Guntur City 4 km from Guntur Municipality office. It has 500 strength studying both Physical and Biological Sciences as well as Arts groups. (*See Figure 3.3 on next page*)

Best and Kann (1992) stated "a population is any group of individuals that have one or more characteristics in common and are of interest to the researcher." The population for the present study was comprised of adolescent girls studying in first and second year intermediate, belonging to Junior Colleges for Girls in Guntur District of Andhra Pradesh. There are 20 Junior Colleges for Girls in Guntur district.

According to Polit and Hungler (1995) a sample is a small proportion of a population selected for observation and analysis. Bhaduri and Farell (1981) have defined Sampling

Figure 3.2
Map of Andhra Pradesh State

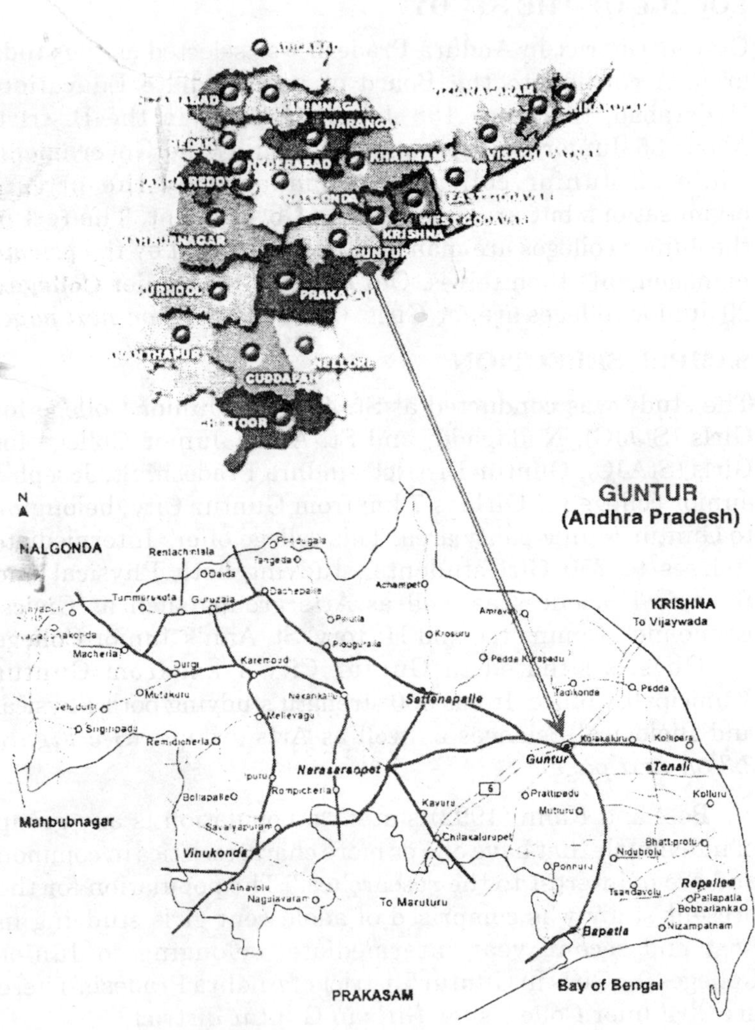

Figure 3.3
Sample Selection

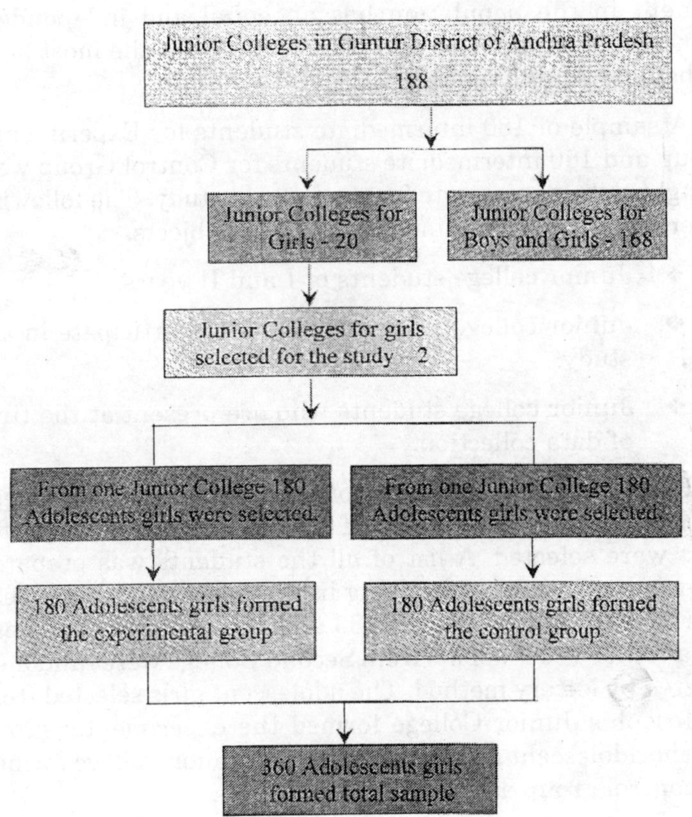

is the representative of those critical characteristics which the investigator plans to study. Sampling is the process of selecting a portion of the entire population. The investigator decided to use the random sampling technique for the present study. The random sampling is the one in, which each element in the population has an equal and independent chance of being selected and which makes for the most basic probability sampling design.

A sample of 180 intermediate students for Experimental Group and 180 intermediate students for Control Group were thought to be appropriate for the present study. The following criteria were kept in mind to select the subjects.

- ❖ Junior college students of I and II years.
- ❖ Junior college students willing to participate in the study.
- ❖ Junior college students who are present at the time of data collection.

From 750 adolescent girls of St. Joseph's Junior College and from 500 adolescent girls of St. Ann's Junior Colleges for Girls were selected. A list of all the students was prepared separately of students studying in first year and second year intermediate. From this list 180 students from First College and another 180 students from Second College were randomly selected by lottery method. The adolescent girls selected from St. Joseph's Junior College formed the experimental group and the adolescent girls from St. Ann's Junior College formed the control group as shown in Figure 3. 3.

SELECTION OF VARIABLES

The researcher after a thorough review of literature and discussion held with the experts conversant with the topic selected the variables for inclusion in the present study.

Independent Variables

1. **Age:** The chronological age of the subjects in completed years was taken as their age from the junior college admission records.

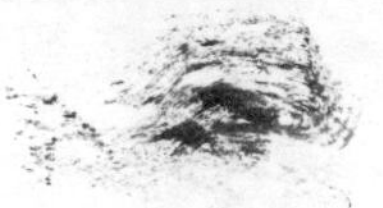

2. **Year of study:** Adolescent girls studying in Intermediate first and second years were included in the study.
3. **Area of residence:** It refers to the place of residence of the subjects *viz.*, urban and rural areas.
4. **Religion:** It refers to the religious faith practised by the subjects, which may have influence on their access to AIDS information.
5. **Caste:** It refers to the social order of the respondents in the society in which they live and grow. Caste status may have an influence on the subjects' level of understanding and perception.
6. **Type of Family:** The type of family determines the subjects' level of interaction and relationship among the family members. The members of the family may have an influence on the knowledge, attitude and practice of the respondents.
7. **Family Monthly Income:** The family's income may have an influence on the respondents' perception of knowledge, attitude and practice. The total income earned by the family in a month is considered as family monthly income.
8. **Exposure to Mass Media:** The sample's sources of knowing HIV/AIDS information especially mass-media was included as an independent variable.
9. **AIDS Education Programme (AEP):** It is a comprehensive teaching programme on HIV/AIDS with regard to the meaning and causes of HIV/AIDS, manifestations and diagnosis of HIV/AIDS, prevention and control of AIDS, its management, role of women/ youth and community in the care of those affected by HIV/AIDS. It includes using of AIDS Education Programme Manual and Electronic Multi-media developed by the investigator for AIDS Education to Adolescent girls. In the present study AIDS Education Programme was considered as an independent variable

as it was an input whose impact was also studied on the dependent variables *viz.*, knowledge, attitude and practice. The detail of the AIDS Education Programme was mentioned in Methodology of the study.

Dependent Variables

1. **Knowledge:** It refers to the Junior college students' range of information regarding HIV/AIDS and their ability to recall this knowledge while responding to the statements on the knowledge scale as evident from knowledge score.
2. **Attitude:** It refers to the Junior college students' expressed beliefs and feelings regarding HIV/AIDS as evident from the attitude scores as measured by attitude scale.
3. **Practice:** It refers to one's ability to perform an activity proficiently (Encyclopaedia Britannica). The term used for the purpose of the study denotes written responses of Junior college students' expressed practices regarding HIV/AIDS as evident from practice scores.

Some Operational Definitions Used in the Study

1. **Evaluation:** It refers to determining the effectiveness of AIDS Education Programme and is measured in terms of significant gain in their post-test knowledge, attitude and practice scores of Junior college students.
2. **Effectiveness:** It refers to the extent to which the junior college students have gained knowledge, developed favourable attitude and adopted healthy practices regarding HIV/AIDS as evident from knowledge, attitude and practice scores.
3. **Adolescence:** Adolescence is the transitional period from childhood to adulthood between age group 10-19 years. WHO and UNICEF use the term "adolescent" for those in 10-19 ages.
4. **Adolescent girls:** It refers to the adolescent girls studying in the Junior colleges whose age is between 14 and 18 years.

5. **Junior College:** Refers to Educational Institutions which offer educational programme at 11th and 12th standards in Andhra Pradesh affiliated to the Board of Intermediate Education. (*See Plate 3.1 on page 97*)

6. **Junior College Students:** It refers to the students who are studying Intermediate first and second year in the Junior Colleges. In the present study the Junior College students are the girls studying first and second year intermediate. (*See Plate 3.2 on page 98*)

RELATIONSHIP BETWEEN INDEPENDENT VARIABLES AND DEPENDENT VARIABLES

The variables selected for the study are inter-dependent having influence on each other. In order to understand the relationship between the independent variables and dependent variables the following figure is designed. (*See Figure 3.4 on next page*)

TOOLS FOR DATA COLLECTION

Treece and Treece (1982) stated that the instrument selected for a research should be as far as possible the vehicle that would best obtain data for drawing conclusions which are pertinent to the study and at the same time add to the body of knowledge on the discipline. Based on the objectives of the study and hypothesis, the following tools were developed in order to generate data.

- *Tool 1:* Questionnaire on Demographic Profile of the Sample Subjects and their Exposure to Mass-media on HIV/AIDS.
- *Tool 2:* HIV/AIDS Knowledge, Attitude and Practice Scales

Questionnaire on Demographic Profile of the Sample and Their Exposure to Mass-media on HIV/AIDS

Polit and Hungler (1999) stated that the common technique used for collection of data is questioning method. A general information questionnaire on Demographic Data of the Students and their exposure to mass media on HIV/AIDS

Figure 3.4
Relationship Between Independent Variables and Dependent Variables

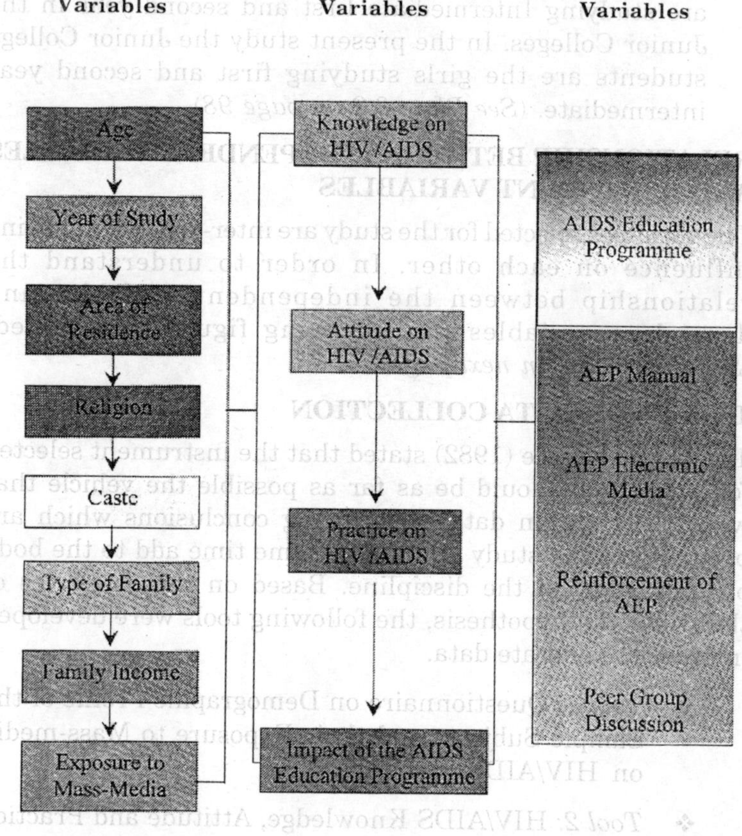

Plate 3.1

Collecting the Data from Junior College Students

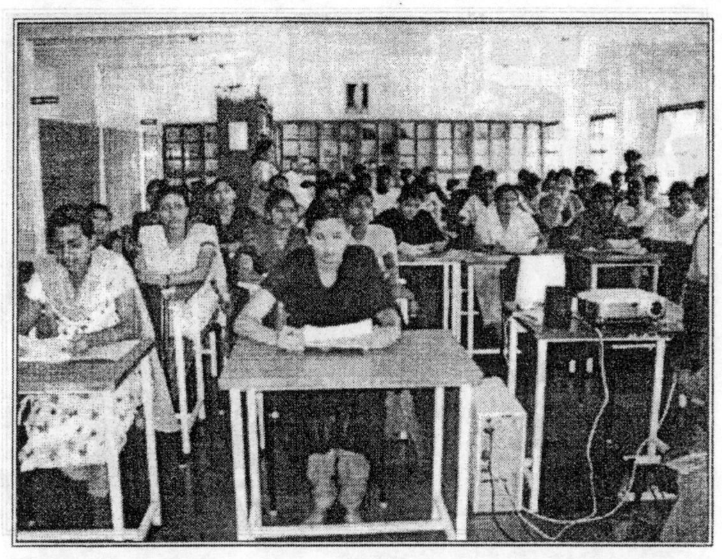

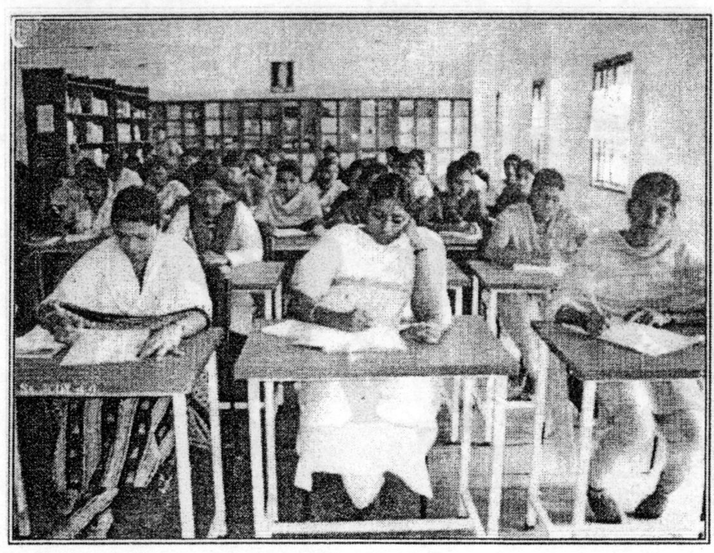

Plate 3.2

Junior College Students During Peer Group Discussion

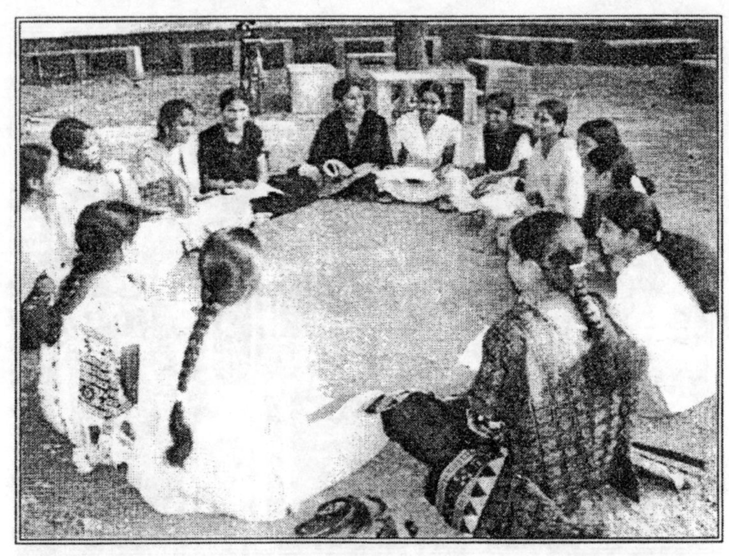

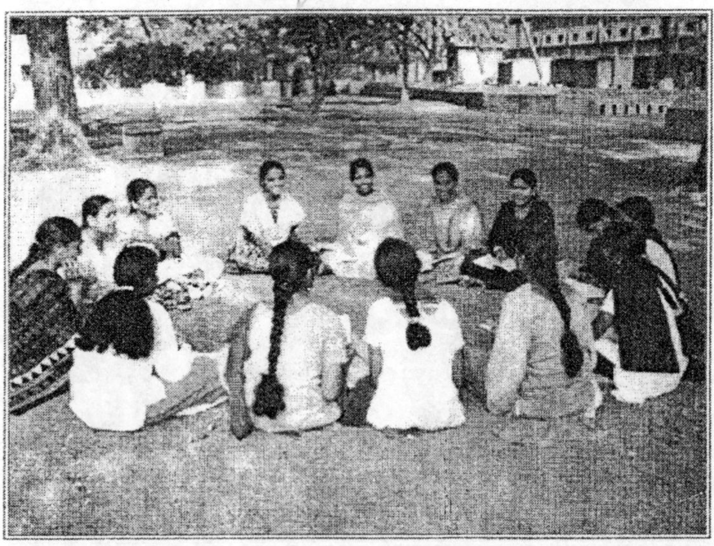

was prepared which consisted of 15 questions of which, 8 questions were related to demographic profile of the respondents and 7 questions were related to their exposure to HIV/AIDS information prior to the present study.

HIV/AIDS Knowledge, Attitude and Practice Scales

(a) ***Development of HIV/AIDS Knowledge, Attitude and Practice Scales:*** HIV/AIDS Knowledge, Attitude and Practice Scales to assess the knowledge, attitude and practice of the students were prepared after a thorough review of literature and investigator's experience in the field. The Knowledge, Attitude and Practice draft scales were prepared and submitted to a panel of six experts conversant with the topic. The experts' suggestions were incorporated and the tools were finalised for the Pilot study. In developing these Scales, the purpose, objectives and specific content of the AIDS Education Programme were considered.

(b) ***Description of the Knowledge Attitude and Practice Scales:*** The HIV/AIDS Knowledge, Attitude and Practice Scales each comprised of 30 items with a *Five Point Likert Type Scale* with five alternative responses *'Strongly agree', 'Agree', 'Not sure', 'Disagree'* and *'Strongly Disagree'*. The positive items were scored five points in case of *Strongly Agree* whereas the negative items were scored five on *Strongly Disagree.* Maximum score was 150, minimum score was 30, and neutral score was 90. Scores 90 and above were considered as favourable knowledge, attitude and practice. The scores below 90 were considered as unfavourable knowledge, attitude and practice. The items on each scale included six broad areas of learning such as meaning and cause of HIV/AIDS, epidemiological aspects of HIV/AIDS, modes of transmission of HIV. clinical manifestations and diagnosis of HIV/AIDS, prognosis and care of an individual with HIV/AIDS, and role of the family and community in prevention and control of HIV/AIDS.

(c) Validity of the Knowledge, Attitude and Practice Scales: According to Treece and Treece (1986), "an instrument is valid, if it tests what it is supposed to test". Content validity of the HIV/AIDS Knowledge, Attitude and Practice Scales was established by submitting the scales to six experts. They were requested to give their suggestions about relevance, accuracy and appropriateness of the items. There was cent per cent agreement by all experts on the content of the Scales. Two experts suggested for language modification of five items from attitude scale and 2 items on Practice scale and it was carried out. Telugu version of the scales was prepared and language validity was established by getting it retranslated into English with the help of language experts.

(d) Reliability of the Knowledge Attitude and Practice Scales: The reliability of an instrument is the degree of consistency with which it measures an attribute it is supposed to be measuring. To test the reliability of the Knowledge Attitude Practice Scales test-retest method was used. The reliability of the Scales was established by administering the Knowledge, Attitude and Practice scales to thirty adolescent girls from a selected Junior College for Girls in Guntur, who were similar to the study population. Time taken by each subject to respond to the scales varied from 25 to 30 minutes. After one month the scales were administered to the same sample. Reliability of the scales was calculated separately for Knowledge, Attitude and Practice Scales using Spearmans' Coefficient Correlation (Rank Order Correlation) to determine the coefficient of internal consistency. Correlation of Knowledge scale was found to be 0.91, Attitude scale

0.93 and Practice scale 0.90. The tool was found to be clear, feasible and there was no ambiguity of language.

DEVELOPMENT OF AIDS EDUCATION PROGRAMME (AEP): AN EDUCATION INTERVENTION

AIDS Education programme in this study was prepared based on programme instruction method of teaching. Programmed instruction can be described as simply a different way of presenting material to be learned different from the way it is organised in traditional lecture and text book approach. Programmed instruction materials are constructed in learning sequences, in which the student actively follows step by step at her, own pace of learning.

Following the principles of programmed instruction method, the AIDS Education Programme was developed on HIV/AIDS which includes: meaning and cause of HIV/AIDS, magnitude of HIV/AIDS problem, modes of transmission of HIV, clinical manifestations and testing for HIV/AIDS, prognosis and care of an individual with HIV/AIDS, role of the family and community in prevention and control of HIV/ AIDS.

The following steps were adopted to develop the *AIDS Education Programme:*

1. Formulation of the objectives and selection of the content
2. Development of criteria checklist
3. Preparation of AIDS Education Programme.
4. Preparation of the First draft
5. Description of AIDS Education Programme:
   - A. Development of AIDS Education Electronic Multi-media
   - B. Development of AIDS Education Programme Manual
6. Content Validity of the AIDS Education Programme
7. Preparation of final draft of the AIDS Education Programme

1. Formulation of the Objectives and Selection of the Content

The objectives and content of the AIDS Education programme were developed based on six broad learning areas. They were: (1) meaning and cause HIV/AIDS; (2) magnitude of the HIV/AIDS problem; (3) modes of transmission; (4) clinical manifestations and diagnosis; (5) prognosis and care of individuals; and (6) role of family and community in prevention and control of HIV/AIDS. The information available on these areas was gathered from authentic sources such as text books, journals and manuals. The messages relevant to the sample was selected and included under the above areas.

2. Development of Criteria Checklist

The purpose of the Criteria Checklist was to validate AIDS Education Programme (AEP) including the AIDS Education Programme Manual in Print and Electronic Multi-media for Adolescent Girls of Junior Colleges. It was prepared based on the literature reviewed and suggestions of the experts in the field. The checklist consisted of criterion statements under the broad headings of: (a) Objectives of AIDS Education Programme; (b) Content of AIDS Education Programme Manual (selection, coverage of all areas, organisation, and presentation; (c) Presentation of Electronic multi media; (d) Presentation of AIDS Education Manual; (e) Language; and (f) Feasibility and Practicability of the AIDS Education Programme.

The checklist had three columns: (1) Meet the criteria; (2) Partially meet the criteria; and (3) Does not meet the criteria. The experts were requested to go through the objectives and content of AIDS Education Programme, AIDS Education Manual and Electronic Media prepared for the purpose AIDS Education. They were to indicate their opinion by putting a tick (√) mark in the appropriate column and facilitate their remarks in the remarks column. The opinions of all the six experts were consolidated and appropriate modifications in the AIDS Education Programme were carried out.

3. Preparation of AIDS Education Programme

The application of technology to education has made necessary for the development of instructional technologies. The technology of mass communication renders possible an amasingly wide distribution of information. Research has shown that a variety of types of audio visual media varying on a concrete-abstract continuum have been successfully used for educational purposes. Audio visual media is used in teaching to provide basis for more effective perceptual and conceptual learning, to increase and sustain attention and concentrating and the personal involvement of the student in active learning, to provide concreteness, realism and life likeness in the teaching and learning situations.

To prevent and control HIV/AIDS among high as well as low risk populations, massive awareness campaigns are being organised through print, electronic media and folk-arts performances. Messages are being disseminated through electronic and print media have achieved greater success in terms of increase in knowledge and behaviour change.

As a part of the study an AIDS Education Programme was planned to impart an AIDS Education to the adolescent girls. The researcher has developed an AIDS Education Programme manual in print and electronic media, which includes power point presentation, audio songs and video film on HIV/AIDS. It was felt that integration of the print and electronic media in the present AIDS Education Programme will contribute to the dissemination of concrete information on HIV/AIDS to the adolescent girls.

4. Preparation of First Draft of AIDS Education Programme

The first draft of AIDS Education Programme was developed keeping in mind the objectives, criterion checklist, literature reviewed, and opinion of experts. The literacy level of the sample, simple and easily comprehensible style, method of teaching, relevance of teaching aids and the attention span of the learners were also considered while preparing the draft. The AEP,was first drafted in English and it was divided into three sessions of 60 minutes each.

5. Description of AIDS Education Programme

The AEP included:

A. Preparation of electronic multi media: development of Power point slides, audio songs and video film on HIV/AIDS; and

B. Preparation of AIDS Education Programme Manual in Print

A. Preparation of electronic multi media: development of: (a) Power point slides; (b) Audio songs; (c) Video film on HIV/AIDS.

The ability to communicate clearly and effectively is a requisite of modern education. The use of Electronic media in education is considered to be one of the most important sources of social influence and change of attitude and behaviour today. Many recognise the power of the electronic media in shaping the habits of thinking and acting of the masses of people.

The investigator explored various methods of teaching as a means to improve knowledge, attitude and practice of the sample on HIV/AIDS. The following teaching aids were considered appropriate and suitable to achieve the objectives of the study.

(a) Power point slides: A set of 28 power point slides were prepared Telugu (vernacular language) using pictures and content from the AIDS Education material produced by A-P State AIDS Control Society (APSACS) and was organised in logical sequence. Prior permission to use the booklets/charts was obtained from the Andhra Pradesh State AIDS Control Society. The power point presentation was found to be simple, understandable, attractive, relevant and interesting. The Power Point slides 1 to 16 on basic facts of HIV/AIDS were used for the first session of AEP and Power Point slides 17 to 28 on HIV/AIDS control and prevention were used for the second session, based on the content presented in each of the sessions. The Power Point slides were also translated into English for inclusion in the thesis.

(b) Audio-cassette: An audio-cassette was used to provide motivation, to convey information, to analyse verbal messages, to provide drill and practice and to teach a skill. The researcher prepared an audiocassette titled *"AIDS Awareness"* consisting of four songs as per the objectives and content area of the AIDS Education Programme.

Song 1: Meaning of HIV/AIDS.

Song 2: Causes and Clinical Manifestations of HIV/AIDS.

Song 3: Prevention and Control of HIV/AIDS.

Song 4: Role of Family and Community in the care of HIV positive individuals.

The steps followed in the audiocassette planning and production were:

- ❖ Identification of purpose and objectives of the study.
- ❖ Consideration of the audience profile, *i.e.* age, education, background of the sample.
- ❖ Strategy, i.e. type of presentation, number of voices, background information
- ❖ Development of the lyrics with desired sequences, characteristics and the message for the content outline; music was composed in popular folk music form.
- ❖ Rehearsal with singers.
- ❖ Arrangement of audio recording in a studio.
- ❖ Editing of the audiotape by selecting, arranging, mixing voices and back ground tunes.
- ❖ Preparation and package in a suitable format.

Telugu language experts, who validated the AIDS Education Programme and tools, validated the content of Telugu audio songs.

Language experts did English version of songs for inclusion in thesis.

(b) ***Video Film:*** The video is recognised as a powerful media of communication. Kumar (1996) says, education and training, creation of awareness, giving information and introduction, demonstration and illustration are few of the many applications of video.

The video film titled *"Crusade against AIDS"* was prepared and edited to suit the present study. The medium of communication of the film was in simple Telugu language and the duration of the film was 35 minutes. The video film covered the following:

- Meaning and causes of HIV/AIDS
- Clinical manifestations and diagnosis of HIV/AIDS
- Prevention and Control of HIV/AIDS
- A case study of Ajay, Lakshmi and Youth/College students
- Role of the family, community and society in prevention and control of HIV/AIDS.

The steps followed in planning and production video film were:

- Identification of purpose and objectives of the study.
- Strategy, *i.e.* type of presentation, background information, planning for the setting and shooting of the film.
- Development of the scenes with desired sequences, characters and the message for the content outline.
- Editing the film by selecting, arranging the scenes, mixing voices and back ground tunes.
- Preparation and package in a suitable format.

Same experts validated the video film titled *"Crusade Against AIDS"* based on the criteria checklist for relevance and suitability of the content and to give their suggestions. Based on the experts suggestions the film was modified and edited to suit the present study.

Telugu language experts who validated the AIDS Education Programme and tools validated video film also. The researcher translated the Video film into English for the inclusion in thesis.

B. Preparation of AIDS Education Programme Manual

AIDS Education Programme manual was prepared with the content relevant to the topic and collected from authentic sources. It included the content which had been evaluated by the experts, conversant with the subject using criteria checklist. The manual was organised as per the pre planned AIDS Education programme. The manual was titled as an *"AIDS Education Programme Manual"* for youth/adolescents. It has a cover page with a title, followed by foreword, acknowledgement and the content on HIV/AIDS.

The subject content of the manual has been organised as given under:

- ***(a) Introduction:*** It introduces the topic, the purpose of the programme and gives guidelines on how to use the manual.
- ***(b) Sessions:*** The Manual deals with AIDS Education programme. One session was meant for the teachers as an orientation session called pre session. For the students three sessions were planned, each of which was for 60 minutes. Though the actual AIDS Education Programme was conducted in three sessions, one session for teachers was included to orient them and introduce the manual to them.

Pre-session for Teachers Meeting: The researcher conducted an orientation or pre session for teachers handling classes for intermediate students. The purpose of the session was to seek teachers' co-operation and also to coordinate the AIDS Education Programme with the college academic programme. It also creates awareness on HIV/AIDS education among the teachers.

Three - Sessions for Students: The AIDS Education was conducted in three sessions for students.

Session I: (on day one) Prior to commencement of the AIDS Education, pre-recorded audio songs (two) on the meaning of HIV/AIDS, causes and clinical manifestations of HIV/AIDS were played to stimulate the curiosity and interest in the students.

The content covered during the first session included basic facts on HIV/AIDS *viz.*, meaning of HIV/AIDS, magnitude of the problem, immune system, HIV/AIDS and young people, transmission, prevention, progress of the infection, signs and symptoms of AIDS, tests for HIV, misconceptions regarding HIV/AIDS and living positively with Positivity. The content was explained using power point presentation and illustrative lecture for 40 minutes. The session was opened for discussion. The doubts and questions raised by the students were answered in the 20 minutes. Thus, the first session was conducted for 60 minutes.

Session II: (on day two) - Prior to commencement of the second day's session pre recorded audio songs (two) on the prevention and control of HIV/AIDS, and role of the family and community in the care of individuals affected by HIV/AIDS were played to stimulate the interest in the students.

The content covered during second session on the second day included Prevention and control of HIV/AIDS:

- General precautions to prevent HIV/AIDS;
- Measures to be taken to prevent transmission of HIV/AIDS from mother to baby;
- Preventive measures to be taken while handling HIV/ADIS infected blood and body fluids;

- Preventive measures to be taken by self and the partner during sexual intercourse to prevent HIV/AIDS transmission; and
- Role of the family and community towards the HIV/AIDS affected persons.

The content was delivered to the students using power point and illustrations *viz.*, charts for 40 minutes and then the session was opened for interaction. The questions and doubts raised by the students were clarified for 20 minutes. Thus, the second session was conducted for 60 minutes.

Session III: (on day three) A video film prepared by the researcher titled *"Crusade against AIDS"* was projected. Duration of the film was about 35 minutes. The video film has the following content areas:

- AIDS as a problem;
- Meaning and causes of HIV/AIDS;
- Clinical manifestations and diagnosis of HIV/AIDS; Prevention and Control of HIV/AIDS;
- Three Case studies on (i) Ajay (ii) Lakshmi (iii) Youth/colleges students;
- Role of the family, community and society in prevention and control of HIV/AIDS.

The session ended with peer group discussion on the subject for 25 minutes. Focus was given to clarification of myths and misconceptions about HIV/AIDS as the programme envisages inculcation of the life skills and positive behaviour among the adolescent girls.

6. Content Validity of the AIDS Education Programme

The initial draft of AIDS Education Programme including AIDS Education Programme manual and Power point slides, audio songs and video film on HIV/AIDS was given to the 6 experts along with criteria checklist. The experts have validated the "AIDS Education Programme" content based on the criteria checklist and given their suggestions for the adequacy and relevance of the content. Modifications were made as per the experts' suggestions.

7. Preparation of final draft of the AIDS Education Programme

The final draft of AIDS Education Programme including AIDS Education Programme manual and Electronic media on HIV/AIDS—power point slides, audio songs and video film were prepared incorporating the experts' suggested modifications. A Telugu language expert prepared Telugu version of the AIDS Education Programme and language validity was established by translating it back to English.

PILOT STUDY

The Pilot study was conducted to test the clarity of the items, ambiguity of the language, to test reliability and feasibility of the scales; and the practicability of AIDS Education Programme and the feasibility of the research design. Formal permission was obtained from the Principals of selected Junior colleges for girls to conduct the pilot study. Thirty Girls were selected randomly. Pre-test was conducted on thirty students using the Demographic profile Questionnaire and HIV/AIDS Knowledge, Attitude and Practice Scales. The pilot study was conducted for three days during which the AIDS Education Programme was carried out on the pilot study sample. After thirty days a post-test was conducted to study the impact of the AIDS Education Programme. (*See Plates 3.3 and 3.4*)

1. Findings of the Pilot Study

The post-test knowledge, attitude and practice scores of the sample subjects was found to be significantly higher than their mean pre-test knowledge score (mean pre-test 95.53, mean post-test 142.73) "t" 28.84 P < 0.001, attitude score (mean pre-test 94.33, mean post-test 141.73) "t" 28.28 P<0.001 and practice score (mean pre-test 93.80 and mean post-test 140.60) "t" 30.19 <P 0.001. The questionnaire on Demographic profile of the sample, their exposure to mass media and HIV/AIDS Knowledge, Attitude and Practice

Plate 3.3

Investigator Conducting AIDS Education Programme

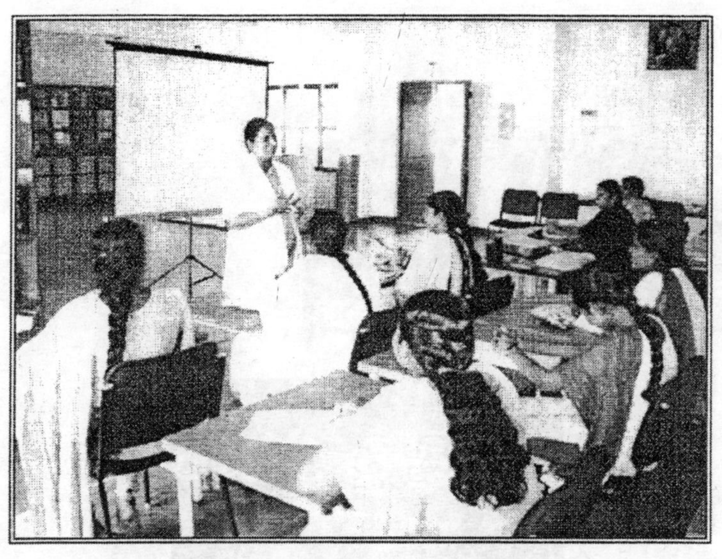

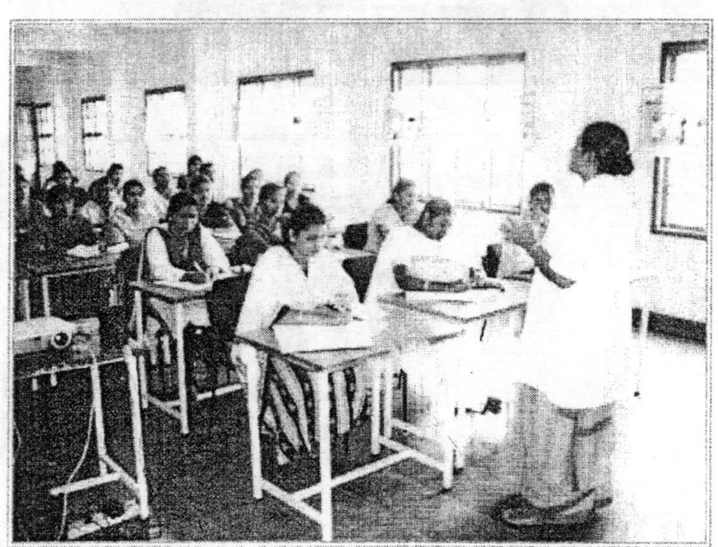

Plate 3.4

Students Viewing Video Film "Crusade Against AIDS"

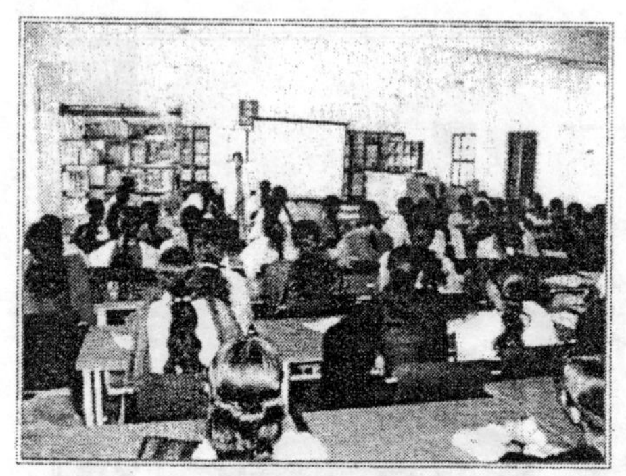

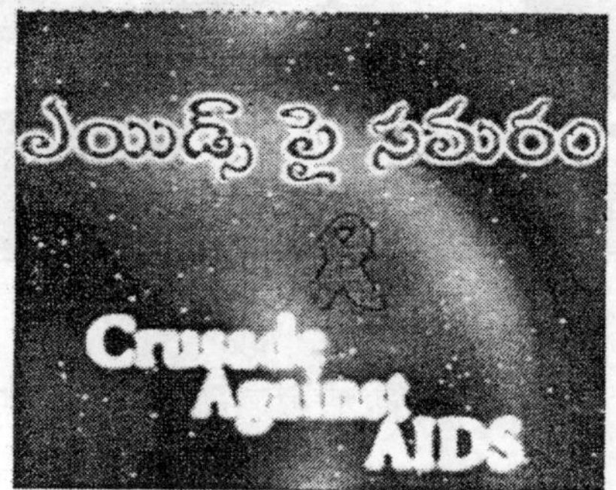

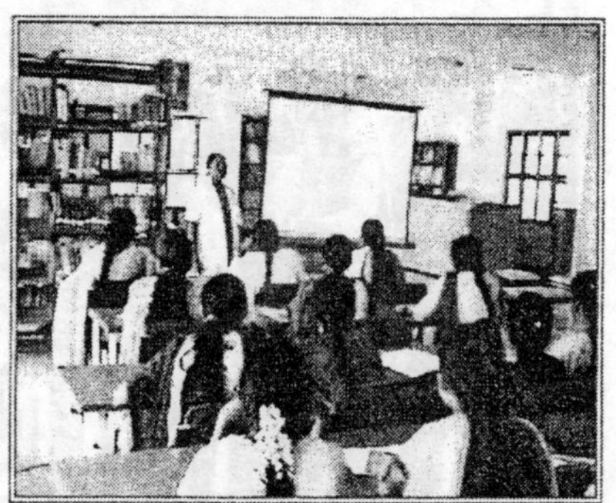

Scales were found feasible. The time taken for each student to respond to these tools was 25 to 30 minutes. The tools were found to be appropriate, clear, and feasible. The research design was also feasible. The AIDS Education programme was also found to be effective on the pilot study sample.

PLAN FOR DATA COLLECTION

Using the questionnaire on demographic profile and exposure of the sample to mass media and knowledge, attitude and practice scales data was collected from the study sample. The AIDS Education Programme was implemented as planned. After a month using the KAP scales the post evaluation was carried out on the study sample. After four months again AIDS Education Programme was implemented to reinforce the educational intervention. After one month of second AIDS Education Programme i.e., five months after the post-test I, post-test II was conducted using the same KAP scales.

PLAN FOR DATA ANALYSIS

The data were analysed in terms of the objectives of the study using both descriptive and inferential statistics. The plan for data analysis was as follows:

- Description of the demographic variables of the sample and their exposure to mass media on HIV/AIDS by frequency and percentages.
- Frequency and percentage distribution, frequency polygon, mean, median and standard deviation, cumulative percentage curve of pre and post-test knowledge, attitude and practice scores of the junior college students.
- Paired 't' test was computed to determine the significant difference between mean post-test and mean pre-test knowledge, attitude and practice scores of junior college students.
- Computing Pearson Product moment Coefficient of Correlation to establish relationship between

knowledge and attitude, knowledge and practice and attitude and practice scores of the sample.

- Computing tests of significance such as correlation, chi-square, regression analysis and t test (r, R, X^2 and t tests) to test hypotheses, to evaluative the effectiveness of AIDS Education Programme, to find out relationship between dependent variables and association between independent variables such as age, year of study, religion, caste, area of residence, type of family, family income and dependent variables Knowledge, Attitude and Practice.

SUMMARY OF THE CHAPTER

The researcher in this chapter presented the research approach used in the study, the research design, the setting, sample and sampling technique, sample characteristics, selection and development of data collection tools, development of AIDS Education Programme, pilot study and procedure for data collection and plan for data analysis.

4

Results and Discussion

This chapter deals with the analysis, results and discussion of data collected from adolescent girls of Junior Colleges. The purpose of analysis is to translate data to manageable and interpretable form so that the research problem can be studied and tested.

The analysis and interpretation of data in this study was based on the data collected through the demographic profile of sample subjects, their exposure to Mass media on HIV/AIDS and Knowledge, Attitude and Practice scales regarding HIV AIDS. The results and discussion of findings were done based on the objectives and hypotheses of the study. All the data were coded and transformed to a master data sheet for computer programming. Statistical Package for Social Sciences (SPSS) was used for descriptive statistics and for testing relationship between variables using tests of significance correlation, chi-square, 't' test and multiple regression analysis.

DATA ANALYSES, RESULTS AND DISCUSSION

The data gathered were organised, analysed and discussed under the following headings:

1. **Section A:** Sample's Demographic profile and exposure to mass media on HIV/AIDS described in terms of frequency and percentages.

2. **Section B:** Description of Knowledge, Attitude and Practice in terms of Mean, Median, Standard deviation, mean percentage, mean percentage gain and frequency polygon of pre-test and post-test KAP scores.
3. **Section C:** Findings related to the effectiveness of AIDS Education Programme, in terms of significant difference in Knowledge, Attitude and Practice scores before and after administration of AEP.
4. **Section D:** Relationship between Knowledge, Attitude and Practice Scores of sample regarding HIV/AIDS before and after AIDS Education Programme.
5. **Section E:** Association between dependent variables Knowledge, Attitude and Practice (KAP) and independent variables such as Age, Year of Study, Area of Residence, Religion, Caste, Type of Family, Occupation and Income of the Family.
6. **Section-F:** Multiple Regression Analysis.

SECTION A: SAMPLE'S DEMOGRAPHIC PROFILE AND EXPOSURE TO MASS MEDIA ON HIV/AIDS

In this section demographic profile of 180 experimental group and 180 control group is described in terms of their Age, Year of Study, Area of Residence, Religion, Caste, Type of Family, Family Monthly Income as shown in table 4.1. The data on sample's exposure to mass media is presented in table 4.2. The frequency and percentage distribution of the sample regarding their demographic profile is presented in figures 4.1 to 4.8.

Demographic Profile of the Sample

The demographic profile reflects the general background of the sample in which he/she is living. Demographic variables also indicate the physical environment of the sample. which may has an influence on the knowledge, attitude and practice of the sample. Hence, an attempt was made to study these variables.

Table 4.1: Frequency and Percentage Distribution on Demographic Profile of Junior College Students

S. No.	*Demographic Variable*	*Control Group (N=180*		*Experimental Group (N=180)*	
		Freq.	*%*	*Freq*	*%*
1.	**Age in years**				
1.1	15 years	63	35	60	33.3
1.2	16 years	70	39	74	41.1
1.3	17 years	47	26	46	25.6
2.	**Intermediate**				
2.1	I year	93	51.7	84	46.7
2.2	II year	87	48.3	96	53.3
3.	**Group in first year**				
3.1	Science (Bi.P.C, M.P.C)	57	61.29	54	64.29
3.2	Arts (C.E.C, H.E.C)	36	38.71	30	35.71
4	**Group in second year**				
4.1	Science (Bi.P.C, M.P.C)	53	61.0	60	62.5
4.1	Arts (C.E.C, H.E.C)	34	39.0	36	37.5
3.	**Area of Residence**				
3.1	Rural	76	42.2	116	64.4
3.2	Urban	104	57.8	64	35.6
4.	**Religion**				
4.1	Hindu	114	63.3	106	58.9
4.2	Muslim	9	5.0	7	3.9
4.3	Christian	57	31.7	67	37.2
5.	**Caste**				
5.1	S.C	48	26.7	54	30.0
5.2	S.T	3	1.7	6	3.3
5.3	B.C	54	30.0	25	13.9
5.4	O.C	75	41.6	95	52.8

(Contd...)

6.	**Type of family**				
6.1	Joint family	30	16.7	34	18.9
6.2	Extended family	9	5.0	4	2.2
6.3	Nuclear family	141	78.3	142	78.9
7.	**Income (per month)**				
7.1	Less than Rs.1000	14	7.8	38	21.1
7.2	Rs. 1001 - 2000	47	26.1	50	27.8
7.3	Rs. 2001 - 3000	41	22.8	22	12.2
7.4	Rs. 3001 - 4000	24	13.3	21	11.7
7.5	Rs. 4001- 5000	27	15.0	25	13.9
7.6	Rs. 5001 & above	27	15.0	24	13.3

Age of the sample

In the adolescent period 15 to 17 years is a crucial age during which the adolescents need guidance and information on matters like HIV/AIDS. At this age they are also quite receptive to receive such information.

Figure 4.1

The Percentage Distribution of Junior College Students by their Age

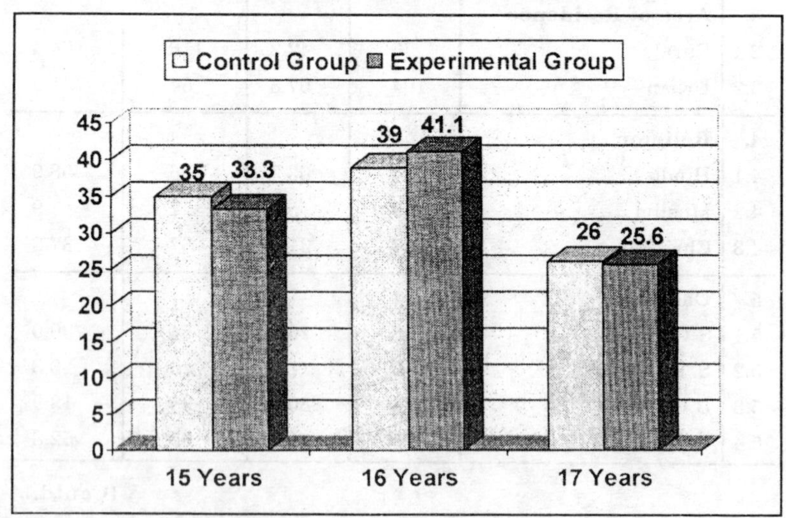

The figure 4.1, shows the data on the percentage distribution of students' age in control and experimental groups. The chronological age of students in completed years was gathered. All the students (100 per cent) were between 15-17 years of age. Majority of the students that is 39 per cent in control group and 41.1 per cent in experimental group were of 16 years age. The data indicates that the target group (100 per cent) belongs to adolescent age group and is potential age for AIDS Education.

Year of Study and Group in Intermediate

Intermediate or eleventh and twelfth class in an educational system is an important stage. The students straight away from school enter a college type of system with increased freedom and autonomy from a rigid and controlled school system. The changes from school to college environment, the physiological and physical changes that occur during this age, create great need for adjustment among adolescents. Hence, this period of transition requires guidance and help in

Figure 4.2

The Percentage Distribution of the Sample by Year of Study and Group in Intermediate

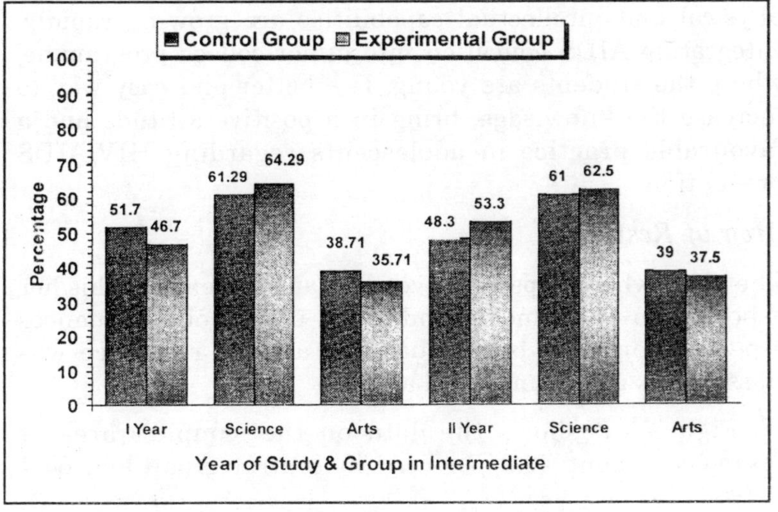

handling some issues, which include sexual health *viz*., HIV/AIDS education.

Figure 4.2 shows data on percentage distribution of students according to their Year of study. Around 51.7 per cent in control group and 46.7 per cent in experimental group were in first year intermediate and 48.3 per cent in control group and 53.3 per cent in experimental group were in the second year intermediate.

As regards to the Group in Intermediate first year, 61.29 per cent of control group and 64.29 per cent of experimental group were studying science group subjects, while 38.71 per cent of control group and 35.71 per cent of experimental group were studying Arts group subjects. In Intermediate second year 61 per cent of control group and 62.5 per cent in experimental group were studying science group subjects, while 39 per cent of control group and 37.5 per cent of experimental group were studying Arts group subjects.

Studies have shown that adolescents acquire ability to process information on critical thinking. and behavioural skills like motivation, persistence, cooperation and team building. Students studying intermediate are in a transition period from childhood to adulthood. Learning is a life process and it is more intense in childhood and adolescence when physical and intellectual capabilities are growing rapidly. Integrating AIDS education into junior college programme, where the students are young, is a better and easy way to increase the knowledge, bring in a positive attitude and a favourable practice in adolescents regarding HIV/AIDS prevention.

Area of Residence

The Area where a person lives has an influence on his/her exposure to mass media and other peer group influences especially on ones behaviour. The area of residence was classified as urban and rural areas.

Figure 4.3 shows the data on the sample's area of residence. About 42.2 per cent in control group and 64.4

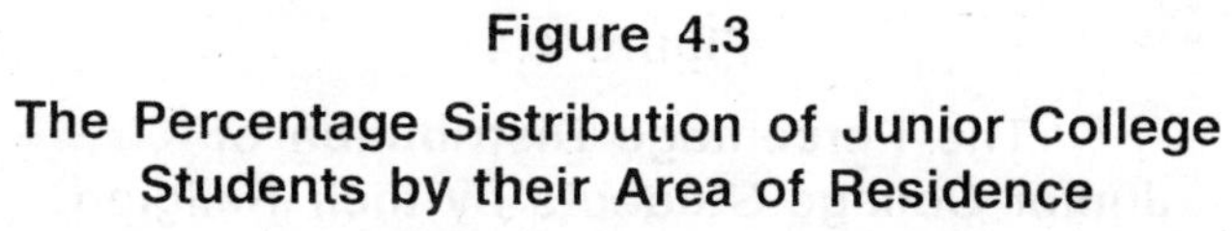

Figure 4.3

The Percentage Sistribution of Junior College Students by their Area of Residence

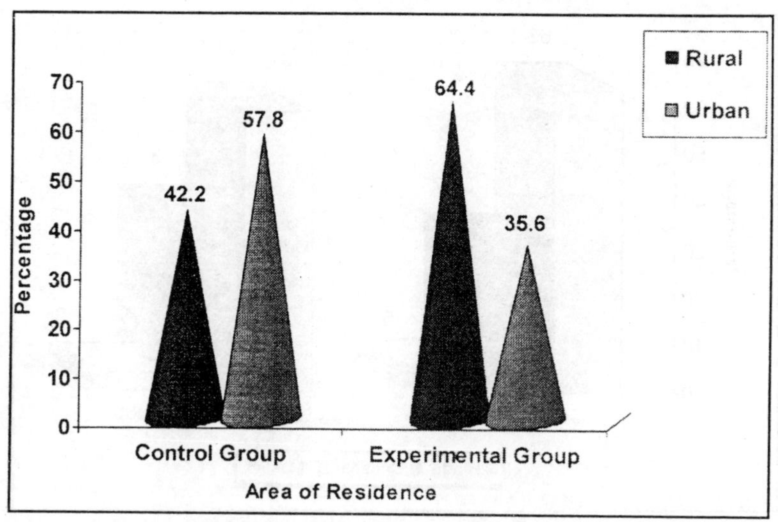

per cent in experimental group were living in rural area, while 57.8 per cent control group and 35.6 per cent of experimental group were living in urban area.

Majority of the experimental group (64.4 per cent) hail from rural area where the influence of mass media is limited, Hence, it was important and necessary to focus HIV/AIDS education on adolescents from rural areas.

Religion of the Sample

Youth is a period of acquiring an identity. Religion is considered as a social organisation where the youth is provided with opportunities for development of good virtues and building up of livelihood skills and contribute to ones behaviour formation and community well being.

Figure 4.4 indicates the percentage distribution of the sample on the status of Religion. A majority *i.e.* 63.3 per cent in control group and 58.9 per cent in experimental group were Hindus, 31.7 per cent in control group and 37.2

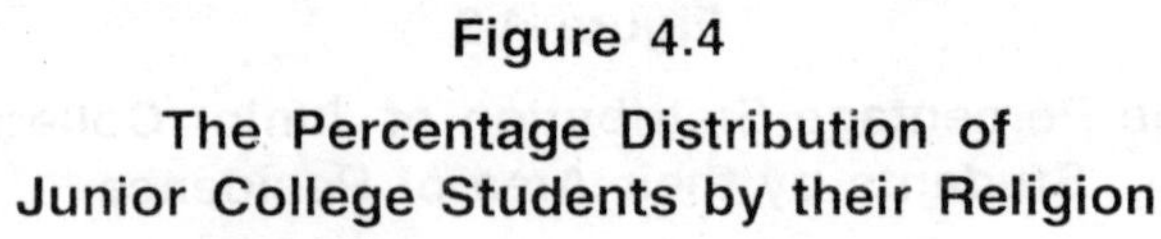

Figure 4.4

The Percentage Distribution of Junior College Students by their Religion

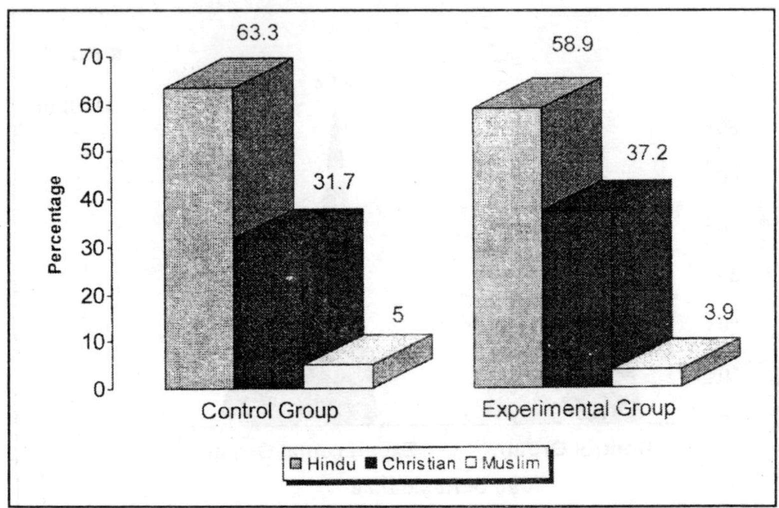

per cent in experimental group were Christians and 5 per cent control group and 3.9 per cent experimental group were Muslims.

Caste of the Sample

Belongingness to social structure in the society is as old as man himself. Caste system has a direct influence on the self-esteem of the youth. Social discrimination, ill-treatment and inequalities of opportunity play a great role on adolescents.

Figure 4.5 shows the percentage distribution of the subjects as regards to their Caste. Data on the caste was gathered based on 4 main classes that are present in the study area. Majority i.e. 41.6 per cent in control group and 52.8 per cent in experimental group were belonging to Other Caste (OC), 26.7 per cent in control group and 30 per cent in experimental group were Scheduled Caste (SC), 30 per cent in control group and 13.9 per cent in experimental group were Backward Caste (BC), while only 1.7 per cent in control group and 3.3 per cent in experimental group were Scheduled Tribes (ST).

Figure 4.5

The Percentage Distribution of the Sample by their Caste

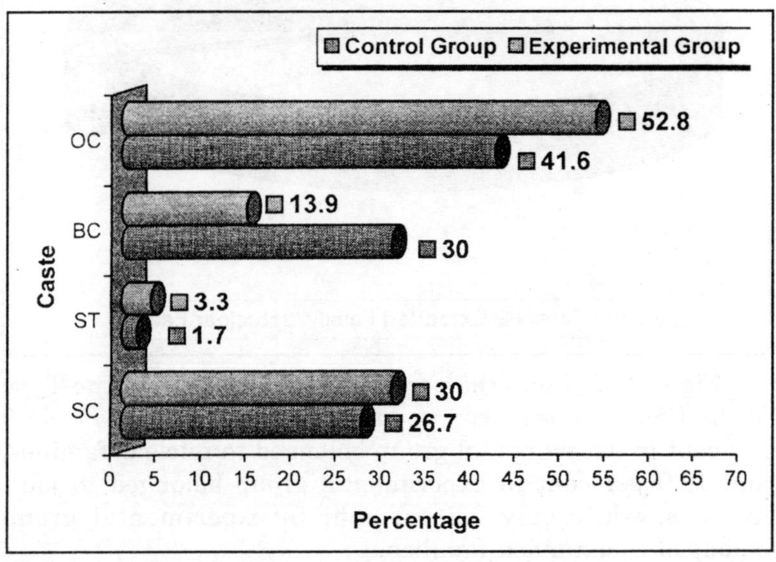

Type of the Family

Type of the family determines the autonomy and freedom of the members towards shaping the future of their children. There is also strong link between the family's female education and health outcomes of the family. Depending on the type of the family the sample's responses were grouped under three main types as joint family, extended family, and nuclear family.

Figure 4.6 shows the data on type of the family of the Control group. A majority i.e. 78.3 per cent in control group belonged to nuclear families, and 16.7 per cent in control group belonged to joint families, while only 5 per cent in control group belonged to extended families.

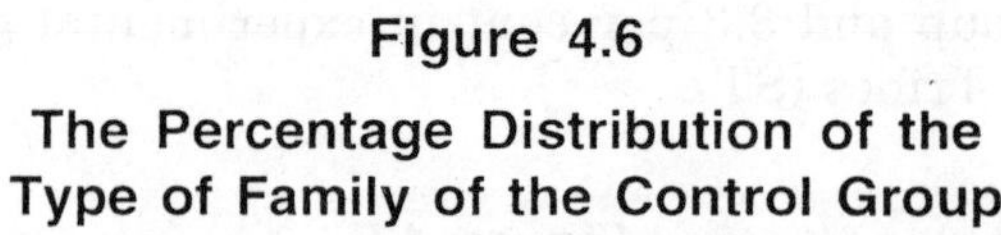

Figure 4.6

The Percentage Distribution of the Type of Family of the Control Group

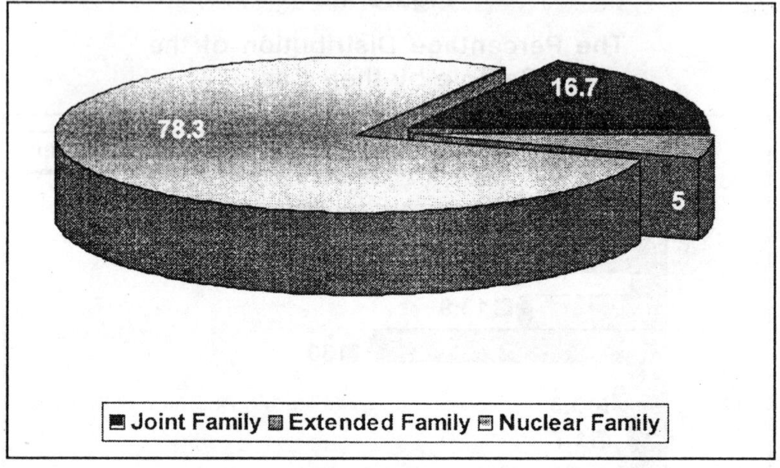

Figure 4.7 shows the percentage distribution of the Type of the Family of the experimental group. A majority *i.e.* 78.9 per cent in experimental group belonged to nuclear families, and 18.9 per cent in experimental group belonged to joint families, while only 2.2 per cent in experimental group belonged to extended families.

Majority of the respondents in both the groups belonged to nuclear families. Family plays a vital role in the life skills of adolescents. Nuclear families in today's society has less time and competence to instill in their children values that are basic and essential for a healthy living and safe behaviour.

Family's Monthly Income

Money earned by the family in a month was considered as monthly income of the family. Based on the family's monthly income the respondents were divided into six groups as given in figure 16 and comparison was made between the control and experimental groups.

Figure 4.8 shows the percentage distribution of the students according to their Family's Monthly Income. A 26.1

Figure 4.7

The Percentage Distribution of the Type of Family of the Experimental Group

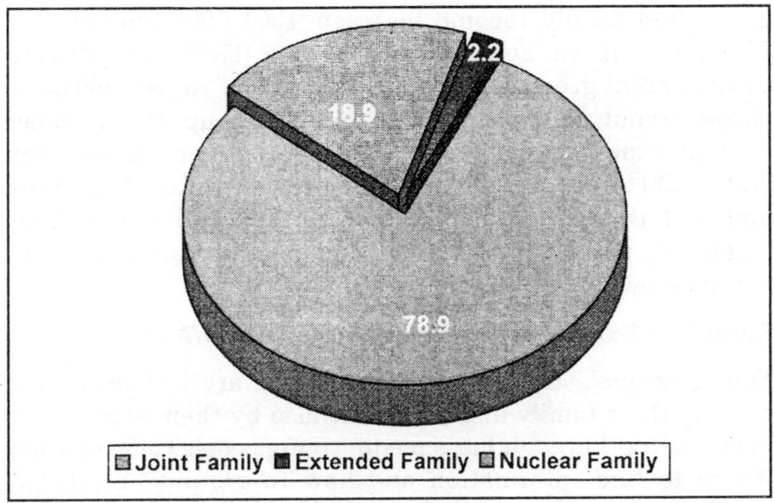

Figure 4.8

The Percentage Distribution of the Sample's Family's Monthly Income

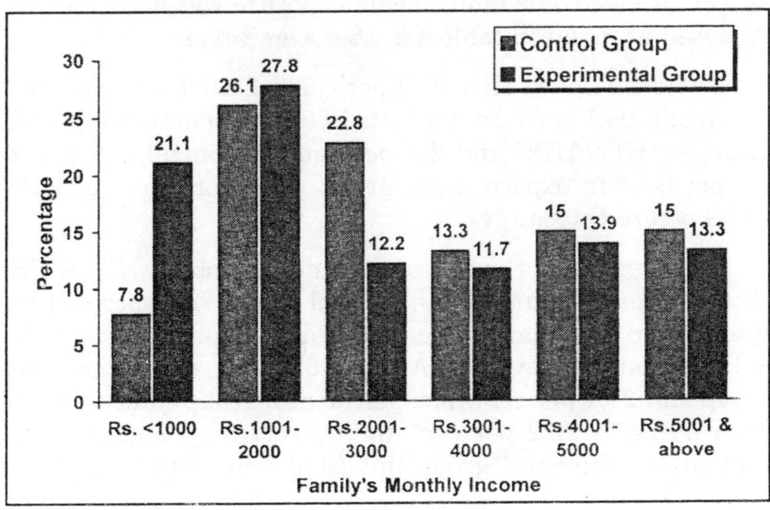

per cent in control group and 27.8 per cent in experimental group had family income between 1001-2000 rupees. A 22.8 per cent in control group and 12.2 per cent in experimental group had income between 2001-3000 rupees, and 15 per cent in control group and 13.9 per cent in experimental group had family income between 4001-5000 rupees, and 15 per cent in control group and 13.3 per cent in experimental group had monthly income of rupees 5001 and above. About 13.3 per cent in control group and 11.7 per cent in experimental group had monthly income between 3001-4000 rupees, while only 7.8 per cent in control group and 21.1 per cent in experimental group had the monthly income of rupees below 1000, which means that they are living below poverty line.

Sample's Exposure to Mass Media on HIV/AIDS

Young people's thinking and behaviour are influenced not only by their family and peers but also by their exposure to mass media. Through mass media young people come to know where to find information and how to acquire knowledge, which helps to develop skills to make proper decisions and how to deal with conflict situations and stand on their decisions under pressure from others. Data on the sample's exposure to mass media both through the printed materials as well as electronic multi media exposure was gathered and analysed as given in table 4.2. (*See next page*)

Table 4.2 shows that 97.2 per cent of students in control group and 96.1 per cent students in experimental group were aware of HIV/AIDS and 2.8 per cent in control group and 3.9 per cent in experimental group were not aware of HIV/AIDS before this study.

With regard to the sources of knowing about HIV/AIDS, 56.1 per cent of students in control group, 46.1 per cent of students in experimental group came to know about HIV/AIDS through television. Around 32.8 per cent in control group and 21.1 per cent in experimental group came to know from peers. A 22.2 per cent in control group and 24.4 per cent in experimental group indicated news papers as their

Table 4.2: Frequency and Percentage Distribution of sample by their Exposure to Mass Media on HIV/AIDS

S.No.	*Variables*	*Control Group N=180*		*Exp. Group N=180*	
		Freq.	*%*	*Freq.*	*%*
1	**Heard about HIV/AIDS**				
1.1	Yes	175	97.2	173	96.1
1.2	No	5	2.8	7	3.9
2	***If Yes:**				
2.1	T.V.	101	56.1	83	46.1
2.2	Radio	19	10.6	21	11.7
2.3	Newspapers	40	22.2	44	24.4
2.4	Signboards/posters	20	11.1	17	9.4
2.5	Health Workers	37	20.6	45	25.0
2.6	Peer Groups	59	32.8	38	21.1
3	**Attended AIDS Education**				
	Programme	64	35.6	59	32.8
3.1	Yes	116	64.4	121	67.2
3.2	No				
4	**Organised by**				
4.1	Government	39	60.9	35	59.4
4.2	NGO	25	39.1	24	40.6
4.3	Anv Other	–	–	–	–
5	**Need to Learn about HIV/AIDS**				
5.1	Yes	180	100	180	100
5.2	No	–	–	–	–
6	**Know HIV Testing Centres**				
6.1	Yes	23	12.8	28	15.6
6.2	No	157	87.2	152	84.4
7	**Know Counselling Centres**				
7.1	Yes	26	14.4	24	13.3
7.2	No	154	85.6	156	86.7

* More than one response

source of knowing HIV/AIDS. About 20.6 per cent in control group and 25 per cent in experimental group stated that they came to know about HIV/AIDS through health workers. Only 10.6 per cent in control group and 11.7 per cent in experimental group indicated radio as their source of knowing about HIV/AIDS, and 11.1 per cent in control group and 9.4 per cent in experimental group could know about HIV/AIDS from sign boards/posters displayed on the roads and public places.

The sample's responses to a question on "have you ever attended any HIV/AIDS Education Programme before" showed that a 64.4 per cent of students in control group and 67.2 per cent of students in experimental group had not attended any Programme on AIDS, while 35.6 per cent in control group and 32.8 per cent in experimental group had attended AIDS Education Programme. A 60.9 per cent of students in control group and 59.4 per cent of students in experimental group had attended AIDS Education Programme organised by the government, while 39.1 per cent in control group and 40.6 per cent in experimental group had attended AIDS Education Programme organised by the Non government organisations.

The subjects in response to a question "do you feel the need to learn more about HIV/AIDS" stated that they all wanted to know more about HIV/AIDS (100%). With regard to their knowledge about HIV testing centres, it was found that about 85.6 per cent in control group and 84.4 per cent in experimental group did not know where the HIV testing centers are located. while only 12.8 per cent in control group and 15.6 per cent in experimental group stated that they knew the places of HIV testing centres. With regard to HIV/AIDS counselling centres, around 85.6 per cent of students in control group and 86.7 per cent of students in experimental group did not know about the counselling centres, while only 14.4 per cent in control group and 13.8 per cent in experimental group knew the places of counselling centres.

From the above, it was evident that the students had varying degrees of exposure to mass media on HIV/AIDS. It was observed that majority of the respondents were not aware about the HIV testing and counselling centres.

SECTION B: DESCRIPTION OF KNOWLEDGE, ATTITUDE AND PRACTICE IN TERMS OF MEAN, MEDIAN, STANDARD DEVIATION, MEAN PERCENTAGE, MEAN PERCENTAGE GAIN, AND FREQUENCY POLYGON OF PRE-TEST AND POST-TEST KAP SCORES

The application of measures of central tendency such as mean and median was to find out the average which represents all of the scores made by the control and experimental groups. As such this gives a concise description of the performance of the groups as a whole. It also enables the researcher to compare two groups in terms of increase in Knowledge, Attitude and Practice scores. As measure of variability the Standard deviation was found to be the most stable index of variability and Hence, employed in the present experimental research.

Knowledge Scores of the Sample

Knowledge about health and health related issues plays a vital in maintaining health and preventing diseases. Enhancing people's knowledge through education and awareness often had an impact on their life skills and behaviour. Young people are more receptive and explorative in acquiring knowledge pertaining to topics like HIV/AIDS. Hence, it is necessary to increase the knowledge of adolescents, which has an influence on their attitude and practices.

Table 4.3: Junior College Students' Knowledge on HIV/ AIDS

N_{RC} 180 N_{RF} 180

Group	*Pre-test*			*Post-test I*		
	Mean	*Median*	*SD*	*Mean*	*Median*	*SD*
Control (RC)	101.54	102.71	6.84	102.0	103.0	7.04
Experimental (RE)	97.06	97.00	8.30	141.5	141.44	3.16

Maximum Score 150

From the table 4.3 it is evident that the mean Knowledge scores (141.5) of Junior college students belonging to experimental group in post-test I was much higher than their mean pre-test Knowledge scores (97.6). The findings also reveal that the post-test I Knowledge scores of experimental group were more homogeneous (SD 3.16) when compared to their pre-test Knowledge scores (SD 8.30). There was no significant difference between mean post-test I Knowledge scores (102) and pre-test Knowledge scores (101.52) of Junior college students belonging to control group.

Kumar et al (1995) observed in their study on teachers that the teachers had deficit Knowledge on AIDS and they also had some misconceptions regarding transmission of disease. Srivastava et al (1997) and Birru (1997) also observed similar findings among teachers and commercial sex workers respectively. Todankar and Sumati (2000) conducted a study among tribal women in Maharastra, found that the women had less information on AIDS and their misconceptions about AIDS were widespread.

Table 4.4: Mean Percentage Knowledge Scores of Junior College students in Pre-test and Post-test I

N_{RC} 180 N_{RE} 180

Group	*Mean Percentage*		*Gain*
	Pre-test	*Post-test I*	
Control (RC)	67.03	68.00	0.07
Experimental (RE)	65.08	94.35	29.27

Maximum Score 150

The data presented in table 4.4 shows that the mean percentage of Knowledge scores of junior college students in pre-test and post-test 1. There was no significant difference found between mean percentages of Control group in pre-test (67.3) and post-test 1 (68) Knowledge scores, as the gain in Knowledge score was very slight (0.7). Whereas in experimental group, the post-test I Knowledge scores increased to 94.35 from 65.08 that is there was a knowledge score gain by 29.27. It indicates that the AEP helped to increase the Knowledge of experimental group on HIV/AIDS.

Bajaj (1993) reported that nursing students had deficit knowledge about AIDS and 10 per cent of them never exposed to information on AIDS. The researcher found that self instructional module on AIDS helped in increasing their knowledge of AIDS and its control and prevention.

Attitude Scores of the Sample

The opinions of youth are influenced by their parents, teachers, role models, peers and mass media. Based on their opinions attitudes are formed. The attitudes in turn influence the thought process, behaviour and activities of the youth. Hence, it is necessary to assess the attitude of the youth towards HIV/AIDS. Positive attitude facilitates learning and similarly negative attitude dissuade youth from learning.

Table 4.5: Junior College Students' Attitude on HIV/AIDS

N_{RC} *180* N_{RF} *180*

Group	*Pre-test*			*Post-test I*		
	Mean	*Median*	*SD*	*Mean*	*Median*	*SD*
Control (RC)	99.37	100.0	6.51	99.85	100.5	6.96
Experimental (RE)	92.81	91.4	10.17	141.19	140.33	2.49

Maximum Score 150

The data presented in table 4.5 shows that the experimental group students' mean post-test I Attitude score (141.19), which was higher than their mean pre-test Attitude score (92.81). The findings also reveal that the post-test I Attitude scores of experimental group were more homogeneous (SD 2.49) when compared to their pre-test Attitude scores (SD 10.17). There was no significant difference found between mean post-test I Attitude score (99.37) and pre-test Attitude scores (99.85) of Junior college students belonging to control group.

Daniel (1995) reported that there was deficit knowledge among Multi purpose health workers regarding HIV/AIDS. Self instructional Module on HIV/AIDS was found to be the effective teaching strategy in bringing about change in cognitive behaviour of multi purpose health workers regarding HIV/AIDS prevention and control.

Table 4.6: Mean Percentage Attitude Scores of Junior College students in Pre-test and Post-test I

N_{RC} 180 N_{RE} 180

Group	*Mean Percentage*		*Gain*
	Pre-test	*Post-test I*	
Control (RC)	66.25	66.57	0.32
Experimental (RE)	62.10	93.51	31.41

Maximum Score 150

The data presented in table 4.6 shows the mean percentage of Attitude scores of students in pre-test and post-test I on HIV/AIDS. There was no significant difference between mean percentage of Attitude scores in pre-test (66.25) and post-test 1 (66.57) of control group, and the gain in Attitude scores was also very slight (0.32). Whereas in the experimental group the Attitude scores in post-test I has increased to 93.51 from 62.10, with a gain of 31.41. It indicates that the AEP helped to bring a positive change in the Attitude of experimental group regarding HIV/AIDS.

Sankaranarayan et al (1996) studied the impact of School based HIV/AIDS education for adolescents in Bombay, India. They observed that such education increased ($p<0.001$) the knowledge and practice about HIV/AIDS and its control and prevention. Meekers et al (1997) also reported that AIDS Education helped in changing the adolescents' beliefs about sexual behaviour.

Practice Scores of the Sample

Application of knowledge and skills is termed as practice. The life skills related to HIV/AIDS prevention and practices related stigma was included under practices. Unless knowledge is used in day today life, there is no use in acquiring knowledge. In order to assess the practices of junior college students on HIV AIDS. a scale was developed, data was collected, analysed and presented in the following tables 4.7 and 4.8.

Table 4.7: Junior College Students' Practice on HIV/ AIDS

N_{RC} *180* N_{RF} *180*

Group	*Pre-test*			*Post-test I*		
	Mean	*Median*	*SD*	*Mean*	*Median*	*SD*
Control (RC)	96.43	96.91	6.77	96.87	97.14	6.58
Experimental (RE)	89.42	88.01	11.00	139.28	139.60	2.45

Maximum Score 150

The data presented in table 4.7 shows that the mean post-test I Practice scores (139.60) of Junior college students belonging to experimental group was much higher than their mean pre-test Practice scores (89.42). The findings also reveal that the post-test I Practice scores of experimental group were more homogeneous (SD 2.45) than the pre-test Practice score (SD 11.00). There was no significant difference between mean pre-test Practice scores (96.43) and post-test I Practice scores (96.87) of Junior college students belonging to control group.

Aplasca et al (1995) observed the effectiveness of an AIDS prevention programme among high school students. The intervention group had higher levels of HIV related knowledge and higher positive attitudes and more likely to show compassion to persons with AIDS ($p<0.0001$).

The data presented in table 4.8 shows the mean percentage scores of Junior college students in pre-test and post-test I Practice scores on HIV/AIDS. There was no significant difference between mean percentages of pre-test (64.31) and post-test 1 (64.58). Practice scores of control group and the gain in Practice score was very slight (0.27).

Whereas in the experimental group the post-test I Practice scores increased to 93.10, from 59.62 with a gain of 33.48. It indicates that the AEP helped to improve healthy Practices in the experimental group regarding HIV/AIDS.

Table 4.8: Mean Percentage Practice Scores of Junior College Students in Pre-test and Post-test I

N_{RC} *180* N_{RE} *180*

Group	*Mean Percentage*		*Gain*
	Pre-test	*Post-test I*	
Control (RC)	64.31	64.58	0.27
Experimental (RE)	59.62	93.10	33.48

Maximum Score 150

The pre intervention Knowledge. Attitude and Practice assessment of Adolescent Girls revealed that all of them had low level of Knowledge, Attitude and Practice on HIV AIDS (about 50%). Peruga and Rivo (1992) also revealed in their study that the level of Knowledge on AIDS and its preventive measures were deficient among women. Bajaj (1993), Muniammal (1994), Daniel (1995) demonstrated deficient Knowledge, Attitude and Practice about HIV/AIDS among traditional birth attendants, multipurpose health workers and female sex workers respectively.

Aplasca et al (1995) identified the reasons for lack of impact of AIDS education on Students attitude as: lack of training to the teachers, need to allow more time for peer interaction and the need to incorporate more intensive student participation.

Kuhn et al (1994) demonstrated the effectiveness School community AIDS education programme. Following the intervention, students' knowledge about HIV transmission, prevention and the course of the disease was greater in the intervention group ($p<0.001$). There was also a significant increase in number of students who claimed to have discussed AIDS with parents, teachers, peers and sexual partners ($p<0.1$).

Klepp et al (1994) also reported the effectiveness of AIDS education school children. Theory of Reasoned Action and Social learning Theory was used to guide development of the educational programme. Following the intervention the pupil of intervention group reported significant higher scores for the following measures than pupil in comparison group: AIDS information, AIDS Communication, AIDS knowledge, and attitude towards people with AIDS ($p<0.0001$).

The Mean Knowledge, Attitude and Practice Scores of the Sample in Pre-test and Post-test I

Figures 4.9 and 4.10 (*See on next page*) present the mean Knowledge, Attitude and Practice Scores of Experimental and Control groups in pre-test and post-test I respectively. The mean post-test I KAP scores of Experimental group (K=141.5, A=140.19. P=139.28) were much higher than the post-test I scores of Control group (K=102, A=99.85, P=96.87), indicating the effectiveness of AIDS Education Programme. The pre-test and post-test I KAP scores of control group are almost same indicating that the low score was due to their non-exposure to AIDS Education programme.

Birru (1997) also stated that planned teaching programme on AIDS and its prevention and control was effective among commercial sex workers in terms of gain in Knowledge and change of Attitude about AIDS, its prevention and control. Robertson (1998) also supported this finding that the HIV/AIDS education with slide lecture presentation was effective. He observed that Knowledge about HIV/AIDS and risk factors in the post-test was significantly increased ($P < .001$) from pre-test status.

Frequency Polygons of Pre-test and Post-test I Knowledge, Attitude and Practice Scores of Experimental Group

A frequency polygon shows the measuring divergence from normal curve. In the normal curve model the mean, median and mode all coincide and there is a perfect balance between the right and left halves of the figure. Frequency polygons

Figure 4.9

Mean Knowledge, Attitude and Practice Scores of Experimental Group in Pre-test and Post-test I

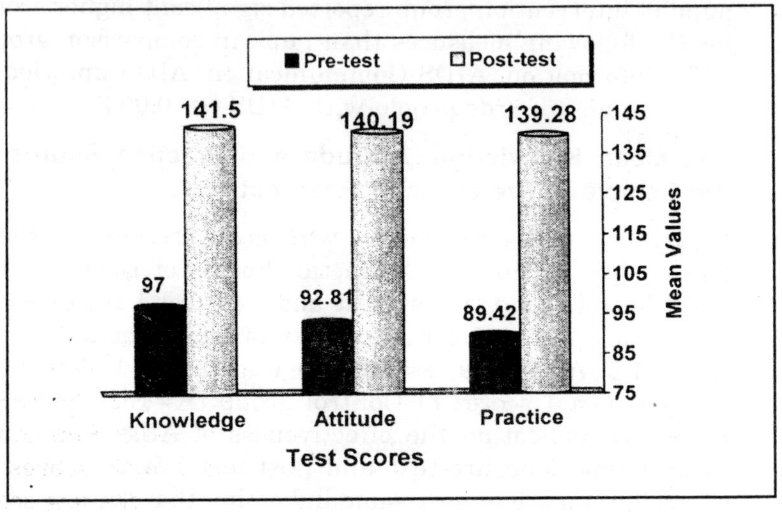

Figure 4.10

Mean Knowledge, Attitude and Practice Scores of Control Group in Pre-test and Post-test I

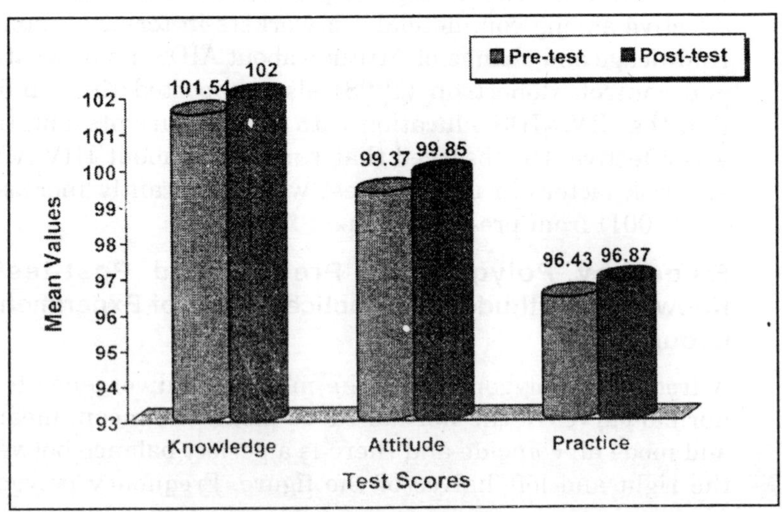

plotted below show the skewness in the distribution. The greater the gap between mean and median, the greater the skewness. When skewness is negative, the mean lies to the left of the median, and when skewness is positive the mean lies to the right of the median.

Figure 4.11 (*see on page 138*) shows the Frequency polygon of the distribution of pre-test and post-test I Knowledge scores of experimental group. The maximum score is 150. The pre-test scores are in the range of 78 to 118 with a mean of 97.6 and median 97. The post-test I scores are in range of 133 to 148 with a mean of 141.5 and median 141.44. In pre-test and post-test I scores the mean is right to the median. The distribution in pre-test scores are negatively skewed. Whereas the post-test I distribution is more of leptokurtic as the distribution is more peaked than normal distribution. The frequency polygon further reveals that the post-test I Knowledge scores are at the higher end of the scale than the pre-test scores which determines the effectiveness of AIDS Education Programme.

The figure 4.12 (*see on page 139*) shows the Frequency polygon of the distribution of pre-test and post-test I Attitude scores of experimental group. The maximum score is 150. The pre-test scores are in the range of 70 to 119 with a mean of 92.81 and median 91.4. The post-test I scores are in the range of 133 to 146 with a mean of 140.19 and median 140.33. The distribution in pre-test scores are negatively skewed, whereas the post-test I distribution is more of leptokurtic as the distribution is more peaked than normal distribution. The frequency polygon further reveals that the post-test I Attitude scores are at the higher end of the scale than the pre-test scores, which determine the effectiveness of AEP.

Figure 4.13 (*see on page 140*) shows the Frequency polygons of the distribution of pre-test and post-test I Practice scores of experimental group. The maximum score is 150. The pre-test scores are in the range of 70 to 119 with a mean of 89.43 and median of 88.1. The post-test I scores are in the range of 133 to 145 with a mean of 139.31 and

Figure 4.11

Frequency Polygon showing Pre-test and Post-test I Knowledge Scores of Experimental Group

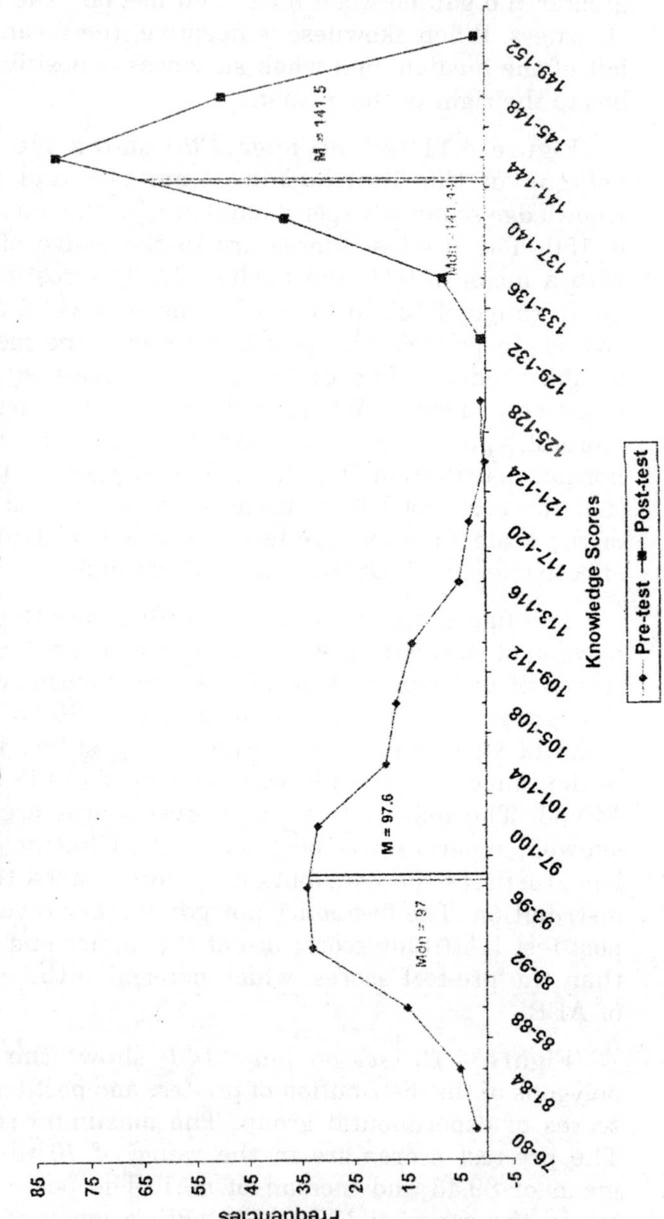

Figure 4.12

Frequency Polygon Showing Pre-test and Post-test I Attitude Scores of Experimental Group

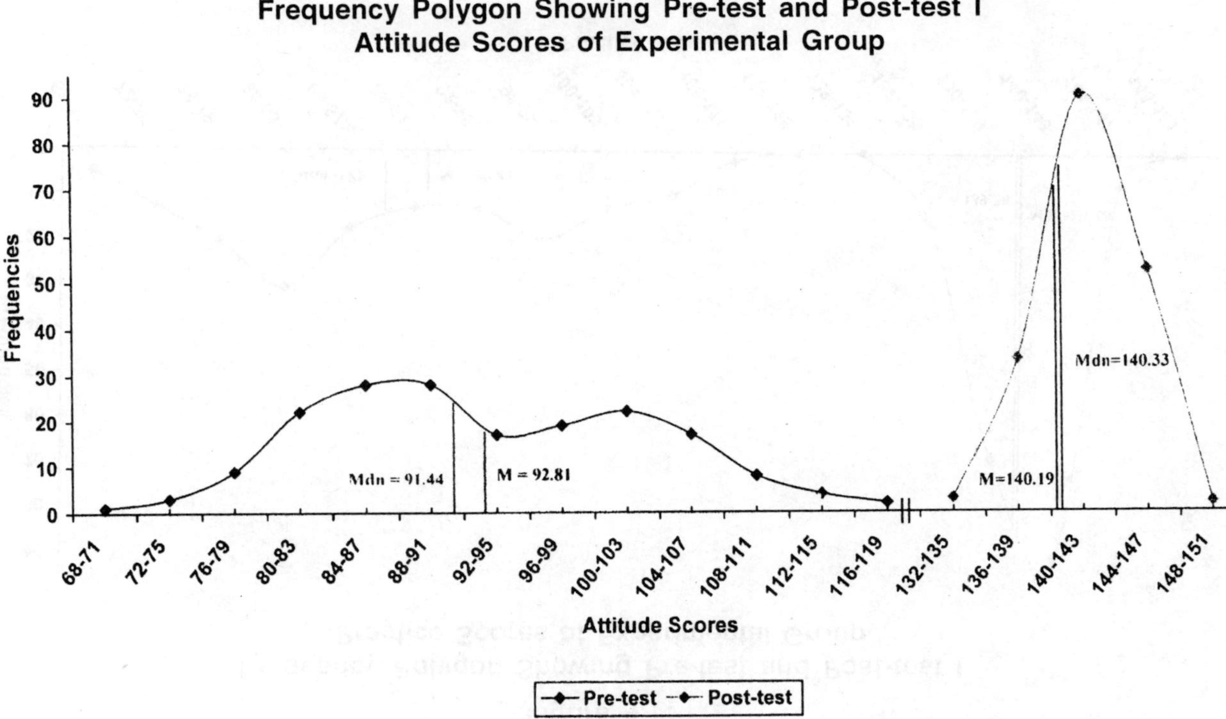

Figure 4.13

Frequency Polygon Showing Pre-test and Post-test I Practice Scores of Experimental Group

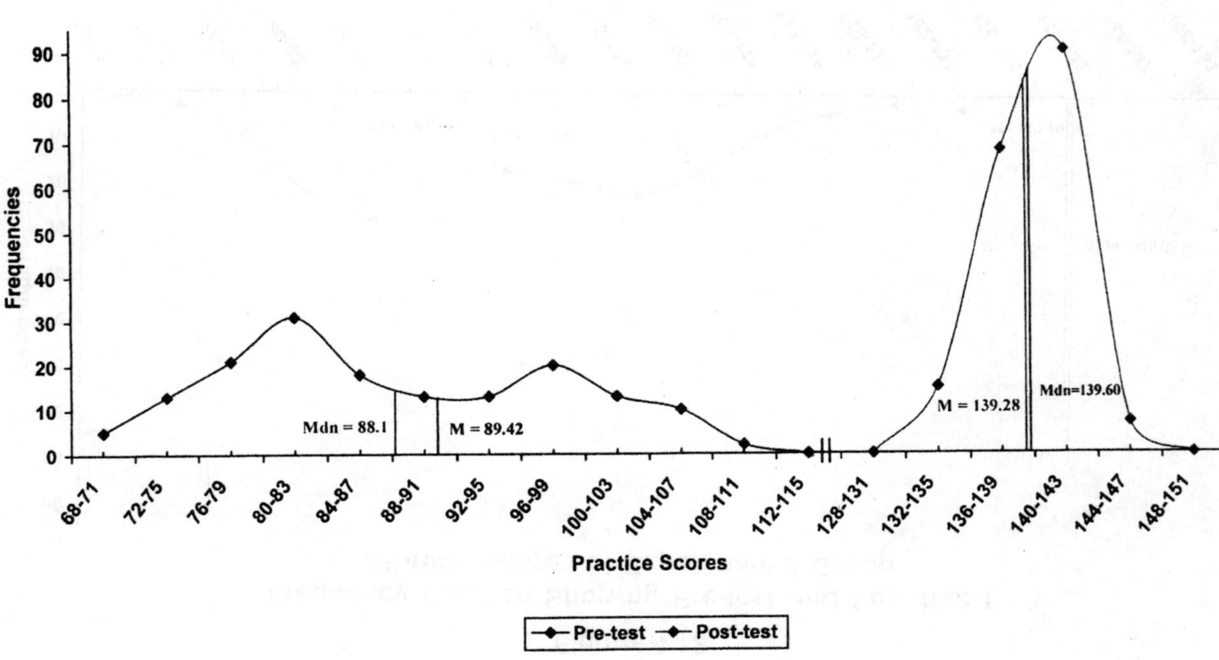

median of 139.60. The distribution in pre-test scores are negatively skewed, where as the post-test I distribution is more of leptokurtic as the distribution is more peaked than normal distribution. The frequency polygon further reveals that the post-test I Practice scores are at the higher end of the scale than the pre-test scores which determine the effectiveness of AIDS Education Practice.

SECTION C: EFFECTIVENESS OF AIDS EDUCATION PROGRAMME TESTING OF RESEARCH HYPOTHESES

Statistical hypotheses testing provides researchers with objective criteria for deciding whether their hypotheses should be accepted as true or rejected as false. Researchers reporting results of hypothesis tests prove that their findings are statistically significant not by chance.

According to Bhaduri and Farell (1981), null hypothesis is necessary to develop a decision procedure for accepting or rejecting a hypothesis. Best (1982) has stated that. the rejection or acceptance of a null hypothesis is based on some level of significance as a criterion. They are of view that 0.05 level of significance is often used as a standard for rejecting or accepting a hypothesis. Therefore, the level for accepting or rejecting the null hypothesis was set at 0.05 level.

One of the most common analyses used to test for significance differences between statistical measures of two samples is the 't' test. In order to determine the effectiveness of *AEP* on Knowledge, Attitude and Practice of Junior College Students, research hypotheses were formulated. These are mentioned in Chapter I. In order to test the research hypotheses, 't' values were computed.

The Difference between the Pre-test and Post-test I Knowledge Scores of Experimental group

To test the significance of difference between means of pre-test and post-test I Knowledge scores of experimental group and to find that the AEP was effective in terms of gain in knowledge the following null hypotheses were stated.

HO_1 *The mean Post-test I Knowledge scores of Junior College Students exposed to AIDS Education Programme will not be significantly higher than their mean pre-test Knowledge scores as measured by Knowledge scale at 0.05 level of significance. (see table 4.9)*

Table 4.9: 't' Value of Pre-test and Post-test I Knowledge scores of Experimental Group

$N_{RE}180$

Exp. Group	*Mean*	*S.D*	*Mean D*	*SDD*	*SEM*	*'t'*
Pre-test	97.63	8.30	43.88	9.20	0.68	64.0** at df.179
Post-test I	141.52	3.16				

Note: Maximum Possible score 150 **P <. 001

The data presented in table 4.9 shows the mean, SD, mean difference, standard deviation difference, standard error of mean, and 't' value of pre-test and post-test I Knowledge scores of Experimental group. The mean pre-test Knowledge score was 97.63, and post-test I was 141.52. Whereas the maximum score was 150. The 't' value was significant at.001 level of significance ('t' = 64.0, P < .001).

Hence, the null hypothesis HO_1 was rejected and the research hypothesis H_1 was accepted indicating the gain in Knowledge was significant and not by chance. This indicates that the AEP was effective in increasing the Knowledge of Junior college students.

Visser (1996) reported that the AIDS and life style education programme for teenagers in South Africa was effective and there was improvement (p <0.005) on all the knowledge scores.

Schuey et al (1999) observed similar findings regarding Sex and AIDS Education among school adolescents as result of school health education. The percentage of students who stated they had been sexually active fell from 42 per cent to 11 per cent in the intervention group (p<0.001) while no significant change was recorded in a control group

The Difference between the Pre-test and Post-test I Attitude Scores of Experimental Group

To find out the significance of differences between means of pre-test and post-test I Attitude scores of experimental group the following null hypothesis was stated.

HO_2 *The mean post-test 1 Attitude scores of Junior College Students exposed to AIDS Education Programme will not be significantly higher than their mean pre-test Attitude scores as measured by Attitude scale at 0.05 level of significance.*

The data presented in table 4.10 show the "t" value computed to test **HO_2**.

Table 4.10: 't' Value of Pre-test and Post-test I Attitude Scores of Experimental Group

N_{RE}180

Exp. Group	*Mean*	*S.D*	*Mean D*	*SDD*	*SEM*	*'t'*
Pre-test	92.81	10.17	47.38	10.63	0.79	59.77** at df.179
Post-test I	140.19	2.49				

Note: Maximum Possible score 150

**P <. 001

The data presented in table 4.10 shows that the mean, SD, mean difference, standard deviation difference, standard error of mean, and 't' value of pre-test and post-test I Attitude scores of Experimental group. The mean pre-test Attitude score was 92.81, and post-test I score was 140.19. Where as the maximum score was 150. The 't' value was significant at .001 level of significance ('t' = 59.77, P < .001).

Hence, the null hypothesis HO_2 was rejected and the research hypothesis H_2 was accepted indicating the gain in Attitude was significant and not by chance. This indicates that the AEP was effective in bringing positive change in the Attitude of Junior college students.

Rossam and Meekers (2000) reported that adolescent and young adult reproductive health intervention in Cameron had a significant effect on several determinants of preventive behaviour, including awareness of sexual risks, knowledge of birth control methods and discussion of sexuality, prevention of STDs and AIDS.

The Difference between the Pre-test and Post-test I Practice Scores of Experimental Group

To find out the significance of differences between means of pre-test and post-test I Practice scores of experimental group the following null hypothesis was stated.

HO_3 *The mean post-test I Practice scores of Junior college Students exposed to AIDS Education Programme will not be significantly higher than their mean pre-test Practice scores as measured by Practice scale at 0.05 level of significance.*

The data presented in table 4.11 shows the 't' value computed to test HO_3.

Table 4.11: 't' Value of Pre-test and Post-test I Practice scores of Experimental Group

N_{RE}180

Exp. Group	*Mean*	*S.D*	*Mean D*	*SDD*	*SEM*	*'t'*
Pre-test	89.43	11.00	49.86	11.79	0.89	56.79* at df.179
Post-test 1	139.29	2.45				

Note: Maximum Possible score 150 **P <.001

The data presented in table 4.11 shows that the mean, SD, mean difference, standard deviation difference, standard error of mean, and 't' value of pre-test and post-test I Practice scores of Experimental group. The mean pre-test Practice score was 89.43. and post-test I score was 139.29. Whereas the maximum score was 150. The 't' value was significant at .001 level of significance ('t' = 56.79. P < .001).

Hence, the null hypothesis HO_3 was rejected and the research hypothesis H_3 was accepted, indicating the gain in Practice was significant and not by chance. This indicates that the AEP was effective in bringing positive change in the Practice of Junior college students.

The findings of the present study revealed that there was a significant difference in the pre-test and post-test I Knowledge, Attitude and Practice scores of Junior College students, who had AIDS Education at .001 level of significance Knowledge ('t' = 66.50 P < .001) Attitude ('t' = 59.77, P < .001) and Practice ('t' = 56.79, P < .001). The mean difference between pre-test and post-test I scores, for Knowledge was 43.89. Attitude was 47.38 and for Practice was 49.86. This indicates that the planned AEP was significantly effective in increasing the Knowledge, bringing positive Attitude and favourable Practice among Junior College Students on HIV/AIDS.

Dutta (1993) in her study revealed that there was an over all increase in Knowledge of health workers on AIDS ranging from 7.7 per cent pre training to 51.4 per cent post training with desirable level of Knowledge and awareness by the use of planned orientation training programme. Bajaj (1993) and Daniel (1995) in their studies observed among Students and health workers' respectively, that the Knowledge, Attitude and Practice levels on AIDS increased after the administration of planned health education on AIDS. Muniammal (1994) and Kuhn et al (1994) support this finding.

The Difference between Control Group and Experimental Groups with Regard to Knowledge on HIV/AIDS

To test the significance of difference between mean gain in Knowledge scores of the experimental and control group, the following null hypothesis was stated:

HO$_4$ *The mean gain in Knowledge scores of Junior college students exposed to AIDS Education Programme will not be significantly higher than the mean gain in Knowledge scores of those who are not exposed to AEP as measured by Knowledge scale at 0.05 level of significance.*

Modified mean gain score was considered for testing this hypothesis. According to Guigan (1969), a modified gain score takes into account the amount of Knowledge that the subjects had prior to their study of experimental material. The experimental material in the present study was AEP. The modified gain score is a ratio of the amount actually learned to the amount that could possibly be learned. It is the ratio of actual gain in Knowledge score to possible gain in Knowledge score.

$$\text{ModifiedGain} = \text{ActualGain}\ \frac{\text{ActualGain}}{\text{Possible Gain}} = \frac{\text{Mean Posttest Score} - \text{Mean Pretest Score}}{\text{Max. Possible Score} - \text{Mean Pretest Score}}$$

Table 4.12: Mean, Actual Gain, Possible Gain and Modified Gain on Knowledge Scores of Control and Experimental Groups

N_{RC} 180 N_{RE} 180

Group	*Mean*		*Actual*	*Possible*	*Modified*
	Pre-test	*Post-test I*	*Gain*	*Gain*	*Gain*
Control	101.54	102.71	1.17	48.46	0.024
Experimental	97.63	141.52	43.87	52.37	0.84

The table 4.12, indicates the Actual gain (43.87) of experimental group was higher than the actual gain (1.17) of control group. The modified gain score of experimental group (0.84) was significantly higher than the modified gain score of control group (0.024). This depicts that the experimental group's Knowledge was higher than the control group regarding HIV/AIDS.

The table 4.13 (*See on next page*) indicates the 't' value on the difference in gain between Knowledge scores of control and experimental groups. The mean gain Knowledge score of experimental group was significantly higher than control group.('t = 66.50 P < .001) Hence, the null hypothesis (HO_4) was rejected and research hypothesis was (H_4) accepted. It indicates that the AEP was an effective method for enhancing the Knowledge of Junior College Students.

Table 4.13: Mean, Mean Difference, Standard Deviation Difference, Standard Error of Mean Gain Difference and 't' value of Pre-test and Post-test I Knowledge scores of Control and Experimental Groups

N_{RC} 180 N_{RE} 180

Group	*Mean*		*Mean*	*Mean*	*SDd*	SE_{MD}	*'t'*
	Pre-test	*Post-test I*	*Gain*	*Gain D*			
Control	101.54	102.71	1.17	41.83	4.28	0.32	66.50
Experimental	97.63	141.52	43.89				

P <.001

Migliori et al (1996) evaluated the impact of AIDS and T.B control programme in Secondary Schools in Uganda. The study reported that the over all impact of health education on the knowledge scores was significant at $p<0.0001$ level, and defaulters started treatment after the intervention.

The Difference between Control Group and Experimental Groups with Regard to Attitude on HIV/AIDS

To test the significance of difference between mean gain in Attitude scores of the experimental and control group, the following null hypothesis was stated:

HO_5 *The mean gain in Attitude score of Junior college students exposed to AIDS Education Programme will not be significantly higher than the mean gain in Attitude scores of those who are not exposed to AEP as measured by Attitudė scale at 0.05 level of significance.*

The table 4.14 (*See on next page*) indicates the Actual gain (47.38) in Attitude scores of experimental group was higher than the actual gain (0.48) in Attitude scores of control group. The modified gain score of experimental group (0.83) was significantly higher than the modified gain score of control group (0.0095). This depicts that the experimental group's Attitude score was higher than the control group regarding HIV/AIDS.

Table 4.14: Mean, Actual Gain, Possible Gain and Modified Gain on Attitude Scores of Control and Experimental Groups

N_{RC} 180 N_{RE} 180

Group	*Mean*		*Actual*	*Possible*	*Modified*
	Pre-test	*Post-test I*	*Gain*	*Gain*	*Gain*
Control	99.37	99.85	0.48	50.63	0.0095
Experimental	92.81	140.19	47.38	57.19	0.83

Mean gain in Attitude scores following the administration of AEP showed that the post-test I scores obtained were significantly higher than the pre-test scores at 0.001 level. This suggests that the AEP enabled the Junior college students to gain Knowledge, positive Attitude and favourable Practice regarding HIV/AIDS. The findings from modified gain scores indicate that the AEP was effective.

Studies conducted by Bajaj (1993), Mandal (1994), Talwar (1994), Muniammal (1994), Barua (1995), Chakravorty (1995), Birru (1997) have demonstrated significantly higher Knowledge, Attitude and Practice in post-test following administration of an educational programme on health matters. Thus, the findings of the present study were similar to other findings related to use of planned education programme. This confirms that the AEP had a great impact on improving the Knowledge, Attitude and Practice of Adolescent Girls on HIV/AIDS.

The table 4.15 (*See on next page*) indicates the 't' value on difference in gain between Attitude scores of control and experimental groups. The mean gain score of sample exposed to AIDS Education Programme was significantly higher than those not exposed to AEP ('t' = 74.88 $P < .001$.). Hence. the null hypothesis (HO_5) was rejected and research hypothesis was (H_5) accepted. It indicates that the AEP was an effective method for a favorable Attitude of Junior College Students regarding HIV/AIDS.

Table 4.15: Mean, Mean Difference, Standard Deviation Difference, Standard Error of Mean Gain Difference and 't' value of Pre-test and Post-test I Attitude scores of Control and Experimental Groups

N_{RC} 180 N_{RE} 180

Group	*Mean*		*Mean*	*Mean*	*SDd*	SE_{MD}	't'
	Pre-test	*Post-test I*	*Gain*	*Gain*	*Gain*		
Control	99.37	99.85	0.48	46.9	6.55	0.49	74.88
Experimental	92.81	140.91	47.38				

P <.001

The Difference between Control Group and Experimental Group with Regard to Practice on HIV/AIDS

To test the significance of difference between mean gain in Practice scores of the experimental and control group, the following null hypothesis was stated.

HO_6 *The mean gain in Practice score of Junior college students exposed to AIDS Education Programme will not be significantly higher than the mean gain in Practice scores of those who are not exposed to AEP as measured by Practice scale at 0.05 level of significance.*

Table 4.16: Mean, Actual gain, Possible Gain and Modified Gain on Practice Scores of Control and Experimental Groups

N_{RC} 180 N_{RE} 180

Group	*Mean*		*Actual*	*Possible*	*Modified*
	Pre-test	*Post-test*	*Gain*	*Gain*	*Gain*
Control	96.43	96.87	0.44	53.57	0.0082
Experimental	89.42	139.28	49.86	60.58	0.82

The table 4.16, indicates the Actual gain (49.86) in Practice scores of experimental group higher than the actual gain (0.44) in Practice scores of control group. The modified gain Practice score of experimental group (0.82) was significantly higher than the modified gain Practice score of control group (0.0082). This depicts that the experimental group's Practice was higher than the control group regarding HIV/AIDS.

Table 4.17: Mean, Mean Difference, Standard Deviation Difference, Standard Error of Mean Gain Difference and 't' value of Pre-test and Post-test I Practice scores of Control and Experimental Groups

N_{RC} 180 N_{RE} 180

Group	*Mean*		*Mean*	*Mean*	*SDd*	SE_{MD}	*'t'*
	Pre-test	*Post-test I*	*Gain*	*Gain*	*Gain*		
Control	96.43	96.87	0.44	49.42	5.86	0.44	74.38
Experimental	89.42	139.28	49.86				

P <.001

The table 4.17, indicates the 't" value on gain between Practice scores of control and experimental groups. The mean gain score of sample exposed to AIDS Education Programme was significantly higher than those not exposed to AEP ('t' = 74.38 P < .001). Hence, the null hypothesis (HO_6) was rejected and research hypothesis was (H_6) accepted. It indicates that the AEP was an effective method for a favorable Attitude of Junior College Students regarding HIV/AIDS.

The AIDS epidemic in women and Adolescent Girls is overwhelmingly heterosexual in India (90%. NACO, 2005). Since the HIV/AIDS affliction is mostly in the productive Age Group of 14 to 40, this study on AIDS Education was carried out on Adolescent Girls (100%) who are all between 15 to 17 years of age. Adolescent Girls are more vulnerable to HIV infection due to biological. economical. social and cultural factors. This study aimed at increasing the knowledge, enhancing positive attitude towards a favorable practice regarding HIV/AIDS among adolescent girls, also tried to empower them, so that they are able to learn life skills related to sexual health and behaviour.

SECTION D: RELATIONSHIP BETWEEN KNOWLEDGE. ATTITUDE AND PRACTICE SCORES OF EXPERIMENTAL GROUP REGARDING HIV/AIDS BEFORE AND AFTER AIDS EDUCATION PROGRAMME

Pearson's product-moment correlation is a parametric test used to determine relationships among variables, Bivariate correlation measures the extent of relationships among variables. Correlation analysis provides two pieces of information about the data: the nature of a relationship (positive or negative) between the two variables and the magnitude of (strength) of the relationship.

Relationship between AIDS Knowledge and Attitude of the Experimental Group

In order to find relationship between Knowledge and Attitude and to test the significance of the coefficient of correlation between the Knowledge and Attitude the following hypothesis was stated:

H_7 *There will be a significant relationship between Knowledge and Attitude scores of Junior college students before and after the administration of AEP regarding HIV/AIDS as evident from Knowledge and Attitude scores at 0.05 level of significance.*

The following null hypothesis was stated in order to test the significance of the co-efficient of correlation between the Knowledge and Attitude scores:

HO_7 *There will be no significant relationship between Knowledge scores and Attitude scores of Junior college students before and after the administration of the AEP regarding HIV/AIDS as evident from Knowledge and Attitude scores at 0.05 level of significance.*

Pearson's product moment coefficient of correlation was used and '*r*' values are computed between pre-test and post-test Knowledge and Attitude scores. The values obtained are presented in the table 4.18.

Table 4.18: Correlation Coefficient between Pre-test and Post-test I Knowledge and Attitude scores of Experimental Group

N_{RE} 180

Test	*Area*		*'r'*
Pre-test	Knowledge	Attitude	.836*
Post-test I	Knowledge	Attitude	.966*

* Significant at 0.01 level P < 0.01

The data presented in table 4.18, shows that the correlation between pre-test Knowledge and Attitude scores was 0.836, which was significant at 0.01 level. The correlation between post-test I Knowledge and Attitude score was 0.966. which vas also significant at 0.01 level.

This indicates the AEP was effective in enhancing the knowledge and developing a favourable attitude. Hence. the research hypothesis H_7 was accepted and null hypothesis HO_7 is rejected.

Relationship between AIDS Knowledge and Practice of the Experimental Group

In order to find relationship between Knowledge and Practice and to test the significance of the coefficient of correlation between the Knowledge and Practice the following hypothesis was stated.

H_8 *There will be a significant relationship between Knowledge and Practice scores of Junior college students before and after the administration of AEP regarding HIV/AIDS as evident from Knowledge and Practice scores at 0.05 level of significance.*

The following null hypothesis was stated in order to test the significance of the co-efficient of correlation between the Knowledge and Practice scores.

HO_8 *There will be no significant relationship between Knowledge scores and Practice scores of Junior college students before and after the administration of the*

AEP regarding HIV/AIDS as evident from Knowledge and Practice scores at 0.05 level of significance.

Pearson's product moment coefficient of correlation was used and '*r*' values are computed between pre-test and post-test Knowledge and Practice scores. The values obtained are presented in table 4.19.

Table 4.19: Correlation Coefficient between Pre-test and Post-test I Knowledge and Practice Scores of Experimental Group

N_{RE} 180

Test	*Area*		*'r'*
Pre-test	Knowledge	Practice	.784*
Post-test I	Knowledge	Practice	.432*

* Significant at 0.01 level P < 0.01

The data presented in table 4.19, shows that the correlation between pre-test Knowledge and Practice scores was 0.784, which was significant at 0.01 level. The correlation between post-test I Knowledge and Practice score was 0.432. which was also significant at 0.01 level.

This indicates the AEP was effective in enhancing the Knowledge and developing a favourable Practice. Hence, the research hypothesis H_8 is accepted and null hypothesis HO_8 is rejected.

Relationship between AIDS Attitude and Practice of the Experimental Group

In order to find relationship between Attitude and Practice and to test the significance of the coefficient of correlation between the Attitude and Practice scores the following hypothesis was stated:

H_9 *There will be a significant relationship between Attitude and Practice scores of Junior college students before and after the administration of AEP regarding HIV/AIDS as evident from Attitude and Practice scores at 0.05 level of significance.*

The following null hypothesis was stated in order to test the significance of the co-efficient of correlation between the Attitude and Practice scores.

***HO*$_9$** *There will be no significant relationship between Attitude scores and Practice scores of Junior college students before and after the administration of the AEP regarding HIV/AIDS as evident from Attitude and Practice scores at 0.05 level of significance.*

Pearson's product moment coefficient of correlation was used and '*r*' values are computed between pre-test and post-test I Attitude and Practice scores. The values obtained are presented in table 4.20.

Table 4.20: Correlation Coefficient between Pre-test and Post-test I Attitude and Practice Scores of Experimental Group

N_{RE} 180

Test	*Area*		*'r'*
Pre-test	Attitude	Practice	.855*
Post-test I	Attitude	Practice	.587*

* Significant at 0.01 level P < 0.01

The data presented in table 4.20, shows that the correlation between pre-test attitude and practice scores was 0.855, which is significant at 0.01 level. The correlation between post-test I Knowledge score and Practice score was 0.587, which is also significant at 0.01 level.

This indicates the AEP was effective in developing a favourable Attitude and Practice. Hence, the research hypothesis H_9 was accepted and null hypothesis HO_9 was rejected.

Thus it was inferred that the increased knowledge and positive change in attitude about HIV/AIDS among the experimental group, helped them in building positive thinking towards favourable practice regarding HIV/AIDS.

These findings are similar to the KAP studies reported by Malik (1988), Fernandaz (1988). Birru (1997) and Kurian

(1998) related to other conditions. These studies supported that the Knowledge played a significant role in influencing the positive Attitude and beliefs and Practices of individuals in the areas of Breast cancer and Breast Self Examination. post-natal care. HIV/AIDS/Adolescent Reproductive health Practices respectively.

Relationship between Knowledge and Attitude, Knowledge and Practice, Attitude and Practice scores of Experimental Group in Post-test II

The studies at aiming at evaluation of intervention programmes usually do not implement follow-up activities to ensure sustenance of KAP. In the present study the education programme was repeated along with peer group discussion. after the completion of AIDS Education Programme I. A post evaluation in the form of post-test II was carried out to study the difference between the post-test I and II.

In order to find relationship between post-test II Knowledge and Attitude, Knowledge and Practice and Attitude and Practice and to test the significance of the coefficient of correlation between these variables the following hypothesis was stated:

H_{10} *There will be a significant relationship between Knowledge and Attitude Knowledge and Practice, Attitude and Practice post-test II scores of Junior college students regarding HIV/AIDS as evident from KAP post-test II scores at 0.05 level of significance.*

The following null hypothesis was stated in order to test the significance of the co-efficient of correlation between the Knowledge and Attitude, Knowledge and Practice and Attitude and Practice post-test II scores:

HO_{10} *There will be no significant relationship between Knowledge and Attitude, Knowledge and Practice, Attitude and Practice post-test II scores of Junior college students regarding HIV/AIDS as evident from KAP post-test II scores at 0.05 level of significance.*

Pearson's product moment coefficient of correlation was used and '*r*' values are computed between post-test II Knowledge Attitude and Practice scores. The values obtained are presented in table 4.21.

Table 4.21: Correlation Coefficient between Post-test II Knowledge, Attitude and Practice Scores of Experimental Group

N_{RE} 180

Variables	*Knowledge*	*Attitude*	*Practice*
Knowledge	1.000	.668*	.478*
Attitude	.668 *	1.000	.440
Practice	.478 *	.440 *	1.000

* Significant at 0.01 level $P < 0.01$

The data presented in table 4.21, shows that the correlation between post-test II Knowledge and Attitude scores was 0.668 and Knowledge and Practice scores was 0.478, which is significant at 0.01 level. The correlation between post-test II Attitude and Practice score was 0.440. which was also significant at 0.01 level.

This indicates the AEP and peer group discussion regarding HIV/AIDS among experimental group was effective in increasing the Knowledge, a favourable Attitude and Practice. Hence, the research hypothesis H_{10} was accepted and null hypothesis HO_{10} was rejected.

This study aimed at enabling and empowerment of the Adolescent Girls of Junior Colleges, who are going to act like change Agents in the health of the community in their future lives. All the subjects in the Experimental Group (100%) in the present study were included in the Peer Group discussions on HIV/AIDS. Park (1996) reports a successful and cost effective plan implemented on a campus of an urban college Peer education programme used student Peers to act as role models to become source of accurate information and support to their fellow students in learning about HIV/AIDS.

The students discussing the HIV/AIDS information among their own Peer Group was successful and cost effective in terms of gain in Knowledge, developing positive Attitude and favourable Practice on HIV/AIDS. Majumbar and Roberts (1998) supports this finding that in their study, AIDS educational programme was effective among culturally diverse women, who participated in the Peer Group discussions about their concerns in their own language and with their friends from the same community.

Thus, it is inferred that the increased Knowledge and positive change in Attitude about HIV/AIDS among experimental group helped them in building scientific thinking towards favourable Practice regarding HIV/AIDS.

Correlation between Knowledge, Attitude and Practice Scores of Experimental Group in Post-test I and Post-test II

In order to find relationship between post-test I and post-test II Knowledge, Attitude and Practice scores and to test the significance of the coefficient of correlation between these variables the following hypothesis was stated:

H_{11} *There will be a significant relationship between post-test I and post-test II Knowledge, Attitude and Practice scores of experimental group regarding HIV/AIDS as evident from KAP post-test I and post-test II scores at 0.05 level of significance.*

The following null hypothesis was stated in order to test the significance of the co-efficient of correlation between the Knowledge and Attitude, and Practice post-test I and post-test II scores:

HO_{11} *There will be no significant relationship between post-test I and post-test II Knowledge, Attitude and Practice scores of experimental group regarding HIV/AIDS as evident from KAP post-test I and post-test II scores at 0.05 level of significance.*

Pearson's product moment coefficient of correlation was used and '*r*' values are computed between post-test I and post-test II Knowledge, Attitude and Practice scores. The values obtained are presented in table 4.22. (*See on page 159*)

The data presented in table 4.22, shows that there was a positive correlation between post-test I and post-test II Knowledge, Attitude and Practice scores of the experimental group. All the correlation values were significant at 0.01 level.

This indicates that the AIDS Education Programme and Peer Group discussion regarding HIV/AIDS among experimental group was effective in increasing Knowledge, a favourable Attitude and Practice. Hence, the research hypothesis H_{11} was accepted and null hypothesis HO_{11} was rejected.

Thus, it was inferred that AEP and Peer group discussion contributed to the increased knowledge and positive change in attitude about HIV/AIDS among junior college students, which helped them to develop favourable practice regarding HIV/AIDS.

SECTION E: ASSOCIATION BETWEEN INDEPENDENT VARIABLES SUCH AS AGE, YEAR OF STUDY, AREA OF RESIDENCE, RELIGION, CASTE, TYPE OF FAMILY, AND INCOME OF THE FAMILY AND DEPENDENT VARIABLES KNOWLEDGE, ATTITUDE AND PRACTICE

To determine the significant association between pre-test Knowledge, Attitude and Practice scores and selected variables a Chi-square was computed.

The chi-square (X2) statistic is a nonparametric test used when there are categories of data and hypotheses about the proportions of cases that fall into the various categories. The chi-square test of independence determines whether two variables are independent or associated.

To test the Research hypothesis H_{12} the following null hypothesis and sub hypotheses were formulated.

Association between Independent Variables and Knowledge Scores

HO_{12} *There will be no significant association between the selected independent variables: Age, Year of Study,*

Table 4.22: Correlation Coefficient between Post-test I and Post-test II Knowledge, Attitude and Practice Scores of Experimental Group

Variables	*Knowledge Post-I*	*Knowledge Post-II*	*Attitude Post-I*	*Attitude Post-II*	*Practice Post-I*	*Practice Post-II*
Knowledge Post-I	1.000	.638*	.751*	.491*	.432*	.312
Knowledge Post-II	.638*	1.000	.521*	.668*	.399*	.478
Attitude Post-I	.751*	.521*	1.000	.368*	.587*	.287
Attitude Post-II	.491*	.668*	.368*	1.000	.240*	.440
Practice Post-I	.432*	.399*	.587*	.240*	1.000	.218
Practice Post-II	.312*	.478*	.287*	.440*	.218*	1.000

*Significant at 0.01 level

$P < 0.01$

Area of residence, Religion, Caste, Type of family, Family income, and dependent variable Knowledge at 0.05 level of significance.

HO_{12a} *There will be no significant association between Age and pre-test Knowledge scores at 0.05 level of significance.*

HO_{12b} *There will be no significant association between Year of Study and pre-test Knowledge scores at 0.05 level of significance.*

HO_{12c} *There will be no significant association between Area of Residence and pre-test Knowledge scores at 0.05 level of significance.*

HO_{12d} *There will be no significant association between Religion and pre-test Knowledge scores at 0.05 level of significance.*

HO_{12e} *There will be no significant association between Caste and pre-test Knowledge scores at 0.05 level of significance.*

HO_{12f} *There will be no significant association between Type of Family, and pre-test Knowledge scores at 0.05 level of significance.*

HO_{12g} *There will be no significant association between Family Income, and pre-test Knowledge scores at 0.05 level of significance.*

Data given in table 4.23 (*See on next page*) shows the computed chi-square values between pre-test Knowledge scores and selected variables; Age, Year of Study, Area of residence. Religion, Caste, Type of family and Family income.

The Chi-square value (23.13) to establish the association between the age of the sample and pre-test Knowledge scores was found to be statistically significant at 0.05 level. Hence, the null hypothesis HO_{12a} was rejected and research hypothesis was accepted.

The Chi-square value (39.2) between Knowledge scores and Year of study of the sample found to be statistically

Table 4.23: Association between the Pre-test Knowledge Scores of Sample on HIV/AIDS and Age, Year of Study, Area of Residence, Religion, Caste, Type of Family, Family Income

S.No.	*Selected Variables*	*Knowledge Scores*		*Chi-Square*	*df*	*Significant not significant at 0.05 level*
		Below Median	*Above Median*			
1	**Age in Years**					
1.1	15 Years	16	44			
1.2	16 Years	20	54	23.13	26	Significant
1.3	17 Years	14	32			
2	**Year of Study**					
2.1	I Year	46	38	39.20	32	Significant
2.2	II Year	48	48			
3	**Area of Residence**					
3.1	Rural	63	53	38.00	30	Significant
3.2	Urban	31	33			
4	**Religion**					
4.1	Hindu	56	50			
4.2	Muslim	4	3	28.13	21	Significant
4.3	Christian	34	33			
5	**Caste**					
5.1	SC	28	26			
5.2	ST	3	3	15.34	18	Significant
5.3	BC	13	12			
5.4	OC	49	46			
6	**Type of Family**					
6.1	Joint Family	17	17			
6.2	Extended Family	2	2	22.16	19	Significant
6.3	Nuclear Family	76	66			

(Contd...)

7	**Income Per Month**					
7.1	Rs. Less than 1,000/-	22	16			
7.2	Rs. 1,001 – 2,000	25	25			
7.3	Rs. 2,001 – 3,000	11	11	9.64	17	Significant
7.4	Rs. 3,001 – 4,000	10	11			
7.5	Rs. 4,001 – 5,000	12	13			
7.6	Rs. 5,001 & above	12	12			

significant at 0.05 level. Hence, the null hypothesis HO_{12b} was rejected and research hypothesis was accepted.

The Chi-square value (38) between Knowledge scores and Area of Residence of the sample was found to be statistically significant at 0.05 level. Hence, the null hypothesis HO_{12c} was rejected and research hypothesis was accepted.

The Chi-square value (28.13) between Knowledge scores and Religion of the sample was found to be statistically significant at 0.05 level. Hence, the null hypothesis HO_{12d} was rejected and research hypothesis was accepted.

The Chi-square value (15.34) between Knowledge scores and Caste of the sample was found to be statistically significant at 0.05 level. Hence, the null hypothesis HO_{12e} was rejected and research hypothesis was accepted.

The Chi-square value (22.16) between Knowledge scores and Type of Family of the sample was found to be statistically significant at 0.05 level. Hence, the null hypothesis HO_{12f} was rejected and research hypothesis was accepted.

The Chi-square value (9.64) between Knowledge scores and Family Monthly Income of the sample was found to be statistically significant at 0.05 level. Hence. the null hypothesis was rejected HO_{12g} and research hypothesis was accepted.

Association between Independent Variables and Attitude Scores

To test the Research hypothesis H_{13} the following null hypothesis and sub hypotheses were formulated:

HO_{13} *There will be no significant association between the selected independent variables: Age, Year of Study, Area of Residence, Religion, Caste, Type of Family, Family Income, and dependent variable Attitude at 0.05 level of significance.*

HO_{13a} *There will be no significant association between the Age and pre-test Attitude scores at 0.05 level of significance.*

HO_{13b} *There will be no significant association between the Year of Study, and pre-test Attitude scores at 0.05 level of significance.*

HO_{13c} *There will be no significant association between the Area of Residence and pre-test Attitude scores at 0.05 level of significance.*

HO_{13d} *There will be no significant association between the Religion and pre-test Attitude scores at 0.05 level of significance.*

HO_{13e} *There will be no significant association between the Caste and pre-test Attitude sores at 0.05 level of significance.*

HO_{13f} *There will be no significant association between the Type of Family and pre-test Attitude scores at 0.05 level of significance.*

HO_{13g} *There will be no significant association between the Family Income and pre-test Attitude scores at 0.05 level of significance.*

Data given in table 4.24 (*See on page 164*) shows the computed chi-square values between pre-test Attitude scores and selected variables Age, Year of Study, Area of Residence, Religion, Caste, Type of Family and Family Income.

The Chi-square value (21.95) to establish the association between the Age of the sample and pre-test Attitude scores was found to be statistically significant at 0.05 level. Hence, the null hypothesis HO_{13a} was rejected and research hypothesis was accepted.

Table 4.24: Association between the Pre-test Attitude scores of the sample on HIV/AIDS and Age, Year of Study, Area of Residence, Religion, Caste, Type of Family and Family Income

S.No.	*Selected Variables*	*Attitude Scores*		*Chi-Square*	*df*	*Significant at 0.05 level*
		Below Median	*Above Median*			
1	**Age in Years**					
1.1	15 Years	32	28			
1.2	16 Years	37	37	21.95	30	Significant
1.3	17 Years	24	22			
2	**Year of Study**					
2.1	I Year	22	62			
2.2	II Year	46	50	29.81	33	Significant
3	**Area of Residence**					
3.1	Rural	61	55			
3.2	Urban	34	30	35.95	32	Significant
4	**Religion**					
4.1	Hindu	53	53			
4.2	Muslim	4	3	16.64	22	Significant
4.3	Christian	35	32			
5	**Caste**					
5.1	SC	28	26			
5.2	ST	3	3	14.99	19	Significant
5.3	BC	13	12			
5.4	OC	48	47			
6	**Type of Family**					
6.1	Joint Family	17	17			
6.2	Extended Family	2	2	16.89	20	Significant
6.3	Nuclear Family	72	70			

(Contd...)

7	**Income Per Month**					
7.1	Rs. Less than 1,000/-	20	18			
7.2	Rs. 1,001 – 2,000	25	25			
7.3	Rs. 2,001 – 3,000	11	11			
7.4	Rs. 3,001 – 4,000	11	10	5.92	18	Significant
7.5	Rs. 4,001 – 5,000	13	12			
7.6	Rs. 5,001 & above	12	12			

The Chi-square value (29.81) between Attitude scores and Year of study of the sample was found to be statistically significant at 0.05 level. Hence, the null hypothesis HO_{13b} was rejected and research hypothesis was accepted.

The Chi-square value (35.95) between Attitude scores and Area of Residence of the sample was found to be statistically significant at 0.05 level. Hence, the null hypothesis HO_{13c} was rejected and research hypothesis was accepted.

The Chi-square value (16.64) between Attitude scores and Religion of the sample was found to be statistically significant at 0.05 level. Hence, the null hypothesis HO_{13d} was rejected and research hypothesis was accepted.

The Chi-square value (14.99) between Attitude scores and Caste of the sample was found to be statistically significant at 0.05 level. Hence, the null hypothesis HO_{13e} was rejected and research hypothesis was accepted.

The Chi-square value (16.89) between Attitude scores and Type of Family of Junior college students was found to be statistically significant at 0.05 level. Hence. the null hypothesis HO_{13f} was rejected and research hypothesis was accepted.

The Chi-square value (5.92) between Attitude scores and Family Monthly Income of Junior college students was found to be statistically significant at 0.05 level. Hence. the null hypothesis HO_{13g} was rejected and research hypothesis was accepted.

Association between Independent Variables and Practice Scores

To test the Research hypothesis H_{14} the following null hypothesis and sub hypotheses were formulated:

HO_{14} *There will be no significant association between the selected independent variables: Age, Year of Study, Area of Residence, Religion, Caste, Type of Family. Family Income, and dependent variable Practice at 0.05 level of significance.*

HO_{14a} *There will be no significant association between the Age and pre-test Practice scores at 0.05 level of significance.*

HO_{14b} *There will be no significant association between the Year of Study and pre-test Practice scores at 0.05 level of significance.*

HO_{14c} *There will be no significant association between Area of Residence and pre-test Practice scores at 0.05 level of significance.*

HO_{14d} *There will be no significant association between the Religion and pre-test Practice scores at 0.05 level of significance.*

HO_{14e} *There will be no significant association between the Caste and pre-test Practice scores at 0.05 level of significance.*

HO_{14f} *There will be no significant association between the Type of Family and pre-test Practice scores at 0.05 level of significance.*

HO_{14g} *There will be no significant association between Family Income and pre-test Practice scores at 0.05 level of significance.*

Data given in table 4.25 (*See on pages 167 and 168*) shows the computed chi-square values between pre-test Practice scores and Age, Year of Study, Area of residence, Religion, Caste, Type of family and Family income.

The Chi-square value (25.44) to establish the association between the Age of the sample and pre-test Practice scores

Table 4.25: Association between the Pre-test Practice scores of the sample on HIV/AIDS and Age, Year of Study, Area of Residence, Religion, Caste, Type of Family and Family Income

S.No.	*Selected Variables*	*Practice Scores*		*Chi-Square*	*df*	*Significant/ not significant at 0.05 level*
		Below Median	*Above Median*			
1	**Age in Years**					
1.1	15 Years	34	26			
1.2	16 Years	38	36	25.44	27	Significant
1.3	17 Years	24	22			
2	**Year of Study**					
2.1	I Year	44	40	29.17	35	Significant
2.2	II Year	51	45			
3	**Area of Residence**					
3.1	Rural	60	56	26.58	34	Significant
3.2	Urban	32	32			
4	**Religion**					
4.1	Hindu	53	53			
4.2	Muslim	4	3	18.92	23	Significant
4.3	Christian	38	29			
5	**Caste**					
5.1	SC	27	27			
5.2	ST	12	3	13.70	21	Significant
5.3	BC	13	12			
5.4	OC	48	47			
6	**Type of Family**					
6.1	Joint Family	12	22			
6.2	Extended Family	1	3	20.19	21	Significant
6.3	Nuclear Family	57	85			

(Contd...)

7	**Income Per Month**					
7.1	Rs. Less than 1,000/-	19	19			
7.2	Rs. 1,001 – 2,000	26	24			
7.3	Rs. 2,001 – 3,000	11	11	5.64	20	Significant
7.4	Rs. 3,001 – 4,000	11	10			
7.5	Rs. 4,001 – 5,000	13	12			
7.6	Rs. 5,001 & above	13	11			

was found to be statistically significant at 0.05 level. Hence, the null hypothesis (HO_{14a}) was rejected and research hypothesis was accepted.

The Chi-square value (29.17) between Practice scores and Year of study of the sample was found to be statistically significant at 0.05 level. Hence, the null hypothesis (HO_{14b}) was rejected and research hypothesis was accepted.

The Chi-square value (26.58) between Practice scores and Area of Residence of the sample was found to be statistically significant at 0.05 level. Hence, the null hypothesis (HO_{14c}) was rejected and research hypothesis was accepted.

The Chi-square value (18.92) between Practice scores and Religion of the sample was found to be statistically significant at 0.05 level. Hence, the null hypothesis (HO_{l4d}) was rejected and research hypothesis was accepted.

The Chi-square value (13.70) between Practice scores and Caste of the sample was found to be statistically significant at 0.05 level. Hence, the null hypothesis (HO_{l4e}) was rejected and research hypothesis was accepted.

The Chi-square value (20.19) between Practice scores and Type of Family of the sample was found to be statistically significant at 0.05 level. Hence, the null hypothesis (HO_{14f}) was rejected and research hypothesis was accepted.

The Chi-square value (5.64) between Practice scores and Family Monthly Income of the sample was found to be statistically significant at 0.05 level. Hence. the null hypothesis (HO_{14g}) was rejected and research hypothesis was accepted.

SECTION–F: MULTIPLE REGRESSION ANALYSIS

Multiple Regression analysis between Predictor Variable and Criterion Variables

Multiple Regression analysis was done to find that there is significant impact of Knowledge test scores on Attitude and Practice tests scores. To find this significance the following research hypothesis was stated:

H_{15} *There will be significant contribution of Knowledge test scores to Attitude and Practice tests Scores at 0.05 level of significance.*

To test the Research hypothesis H_{15} the following null hypothesis was formulated.

HO_{15} *There will be no significant contribution of Knowledge test scores to Attitude and Practice tests Scores at 0.05 level of significance.*

Multiple Regression analysis was done by the statistical Package of Social Sciences (SPSS) to establish the predictive validity of the Knowledge scores. Kerlinger (1983) reports that "multiple regression is an efficient and powerful means of hypothesis testing and inference making technique, since it helps the scientific study with relative precision, complex inter-relation between independent variables and dependent variable and this help to explain the presumed phenomenon represented by the dependent variable.

Step-wise regression analysis procedure defines a posterior order based solely on the relative uniqueness of the variables in the sample. Table 4.26 (*See on page 170*) shows the stepwise regression analysis with Knowledge score as dependent variable and Attitude and Practice scores as independent variables in Experimental and Control groups separately. The data presented in table 4.26, indicates multiple correlation coefficient (Multiple R), coefficients of multiple determination (R2) and its significance (F ratio) for the study.

Table 4.26: Multiple Regression Analysis Between Knowledge Test Scores and Attitude and Practice Tests Scores

Variables	*Multiple R*	R^2	SE_E	*F-ratio*	*Sig.**
Experimental Group					
Attitude Pre-test	.836	.698	4.5754	411.64	.001
Practice pre-test	.846	.716	4.4522	223.01	.001
Attitude post-test I	.751	.564	2.0948	230.57	.001
Practice post-test I	.432	.187	2.8618	40.91	.001
Control Group					
Attitude pre-test	.721	.519	4.8758	192.29	.001
Practice pre-test	.587	.345	5.6927	93.644	.001
Attitude post-test I	.660	.435	5.1542	137.02	.001
Practice post-test I	.516	.266	5.8742	64.87	.001

Dependent variable: Knowledge tests scores.

* Significant at 0.001 level

The table 4.26, presents the values of Multiple Regression. R_2 values are shown in order of entrance in the equation. For experimental pre test Knowledge scores, pre-test Attitude scores was the first variable to be stepped into the regression analysis (R^2 = 0.698) followed by pre-test Practice scores (R^2 = 0.717). For post-test Knowledge scores, post-test I Attitude scores was the first variable to be stepped into the regression analysis (R^2 = 0.564) and followed post-test I Practice scores (R^2 = 0.187)

For control group pre test Knowledge scores, pre-test Attitude scores was the first variable to be stepped into the regression analysis (R^2 = 0.519) followed by pre-test Practice scores (R^2 = 0.345). For post-test I Knowledge scores, post-test I Attitude scores was the first variable to be stepped into the regression analysis (R2 = 0.435) followed by post-test I Practice scores (R^2 = 0.266)

In order to find the significance of R^2 values, F ratios were computed. All R^2 values were significant at .0001 level. Thus HO_{15} was rejected research hypothesis (H_{15}) was accepted indicating that there was significant contribution of Knowledge test scores to Attitude and Practice tests scores.

SUMMARY OF THE CHAPTER

This chapter dealt with the analyses, results and discussion of the findings of the study. The data gathered were summarised in the master data sheets and both descriptive and inferential statistics were used for analysis.

The analysis had been organised and presented under various sections. Frequencies and percentages were used to analyse the sample characteristics.

Mean, Median. Standard Deviation, and Frequency, percentage of pre and post-test knowledge scores are computed to describe the Knowledge. Attitude and Practice of the sample.

Mean percentages, and actual and modified gain was computed to analyze the effectiveness of planned AIDS Education Programme in terms of gain in knowledge, attitude and practice 't' test was computed to determine the significance of difference in knowledge, attitude and practice pre-test and post-tests.

Correlation was computed to find the relationship between pre-test and post-test Knowledge. Attitude and Practice scores.

Chi-square was computed to test the association between KAP and selected independent variables.

Multiple Regression was computed to know to the impact of Knowledge scores on Attitude and Practice Scores.

5

Summary and Conclusion

The education sectors of affected countries play an increasingly important role in the fight against HIV/AIDS. Education has a dramatic impact on the prevention and control of HIV infection and development of a nation. The increasing role of education sectors recognise that a good education is one of the most effective way of helping young people to avoid HIV/AIDS. For these adolescents and youth there is a window of hope, a chance of a life from AIDS if they can acquire the knowledge, skills and values to help them protect themselves as they grow up. Providing young people with the "Social Vaccine" of education offers them a real chance of productive life (World Bank, 2002)

Studies have shown that appropriately trained and educated young peer educators provide effective information necessary for behaviour change through positive influence among their younger peers. Students exposed to school and college AIDS Education can also educate their own peers both in and out of school/college as well as older generations. HIV/AIDS prevention education efforts all over the world aim at youth and adolescents. It focuses on reducing the negative consequences of premature and adolescent sex by promoting sexual health and healthy life styles for young people. The education must deal with the broader context of sexual behaviour and it should be sustained over many years at same level of intensity to hold the attention of youth and public in general.

SUMMARY OF THE STUDY

The present study was an action research which aimed at evaluating the effectiveness of AIDS Education Programme for Adolescent Girls studying in Junior Colleges.

Objectives of the Study

1. To develop tools for assessing the Knowledge, Attitude and Practice of the adolescent girls on HIV/AIDS.
2. To develop and validate AIDS Education Programme (AEP).
3. To develop AIDS Education Programme manual in print and electronic multi media for AIDS Education.
4. To assess the Knowledge. Attitude and Practice of the adolescent girls of Junior Colleges on HIV AIDS before and after the administration of AIDS Education Programme.
5. To study the effectiveness of the AIDS Education Programme in terms of gains in Knowledge, Attitude, and Practice among the adolescent girls of Junior Colleges.
6. To study the relationship between Knowledge, Attitude and Practice of adolescent girls on HIV/AIDS.
7. To study the association between independent variables such as Age, Year of Study, Religion, Caste, Place of Residence, Type of Family, Family Income and dependent variables Knowledge, Attitude and Practice.

Research Design

The present study was an action research in nature and the research design was based on Systems model. The model consists of three phases: input, process, output and a context.

Input refers to target Adolescent girls from Junior Colleges with their background and existing characteristics such as demographic data, their existing knowledge. attitude and practice regarding HIV/AIDS and exposure to mass media on HIV AIDS.

The process included the development of the tools on Demographic profile and exposure of the sample to mass media, development of knowledge, attitude and practice scales and assessment of data using these tools. Process also refers to the different operational procedures in the overall programme implementation of AIDS Education Programme (AEP). The different activities in the process include development of AIDS Education Programme, development of objectives, development of checklist for validation, preparation of the AIDS Education Programme, development of AIDS Education Manual in print and electronic multi media and administration of AEP using the AIDS Education Manual and electronic multi media to Junior college students.

The Output was evaluated by analysing the Demographic profile and exposure of the sample to mass media and the Knowledge, Attitude and Practice gained by Adolescent girls on HIV/AIDS after the administration of the AIDS Education programme.

Context refers to the environment in which the AIDS Education Programme took place. In the present study, the context refers to Junior Colleges for girls, where the target group was living at the time of the study.

Hypotheses

H_1 *The mean post-test I Knowledge scores of Junior College Students exposed to AEP will be significantly higher than their mean pre-test Knowledge scores as measured by Knowledge scale at 0.05 level of significance.*

H_2 *The mean post-test I Attitude scores of Junior College Students exposed to AEP will be significantly higher than their mean pre-test Attitude scores as measured by Attitude scale at 0.05 level of significance.*

H_3 *The mean post-test I Practice scores of Junior College Students exposed to AEP will be significantly higher than that of their mean pre-test Practice scores as measured by Practice scale at 0.05 level of significance.*

H_4 *The mean gain in Knowledge score of Junior College Students exposed to AEP will be significantly higher than the mean gain in Knowledge scores of those who are not exposed to AEP as measured by Knowledge scale at 0.05 level of significance.*

H_5 *The mean gain in Attitude score of Junior college students exposed to AEP will be significantly higher than the mean gain in Attitude scores of those who are not exposed to AEP as measured by Attitude scale at 0.05 level of significance.*

H_6 *The mean gain in Practice score of Junior college students exposed to AEP will be significantly higher than the mean gain in Practice scores of those who are not exposed to AEP as measured by Practice scale at 0.05 level of significance.*

H_7 *There will be a significant relationship between Knowledge and Attitude scores of Junior college students before and after the administration of AEP regarding HIV/AIDS as evident from Knowledge and Attitude scores at 0.05 level of significance.*

H_8 *There will be a significant relationship between Knowledge and Practice scores of Junior college students before and after the administration of AEP regarding HIV/AIDS as evident from Knowledge and Practice scores at 0.05 level of significance.*

H_9 *There will be a significant relationship between Attitude and Practice scores of Junior college students before and after the administration of AEP regarding HIV/AIDS as evident from Attitude and Practice scores at 0.05 level of significance.*

H_{10} *There will be a significant relationship between Knowledge and Attitude Knowledge and Practice.*

Attitude and Practice post-test II scores of Junior college students regarding HIV/AIDS as evident from KAP post-test II scores at 0.05 level of significance.

***H*$_{11}$** *There will be a significant relationship between post-test I and post-test II Knowledge, Attitude and Practice scores of Junior college students regarding HIV/AIDS as evident from KAP post-test I and post-test II scores at 0.05 level of significance.*

***H*$_{12}$** *There will be a significant association between the selected independent variables: Age, Year of Study, Place of Residence, Religion, Caste, Type of Family, Family Income, and dependent variable Knowledge at 0.05 level of significance.*

***H*$_{13}$** *There will be a significant association between the selected independent variables: Age, Year of Study, Place of residence, Religion, Caste. Type of family, Family income, and dependent variable Attitude at 0.05 level of significance.*

***H*$_{14}$** *There will be a significant association between the selected independent variables: Age, Year of Study, Place of Residence, Religion. Caste. Type of Family, Family Income, and dependent variable Practice at 0.05 level of significance.*

***H*$_{15}$** *There will be a significant contribution of Knowledge test scores to Attitude and Practice test scores at 0.05 level of significance.*

Variables

The independent variables were the demographic profile of the sample such as Age, Year of Study. Place of Residence, Religion, Caste, Type of family and Family Income. The dependent variables were the Knowledge, Attitude and Practice scores of adolescent girls on HIV/AIDS. Both the independent and dependent variables were statistically treated.

Methodology

The research design used for the present study was an action research which measured the effectiveness of an AIDS

Education Programme on a randomly selected 180 Experimental and 180 Control Group samples of adolescent girls from selected Junior Colleges of Guntur district in Andhra Pradesh.

A Questionnaire on Demographic profile and exposure of the sample to mass media on HIV/AIDS was used to collect data on sample characteristics and their exposure to mass media on HIV/AIDS. Using Knowledge, Attitude and Practice Scales pre-test and post-tests were conducted to generate the data. AIDS Education Programme was conducted to experimental group using AIDS Education Programme manual and Electronic multi media.

Based on the objectives and the hypotheses, the data was analysed using both descriptive and inferential statistics. The descriptive statistics used were frequency and percentages. mean percentage, mean, median, standard deviation and frequency polygon. The tests of significance such as 't' test and Correlation 'r', Chi-square 'X^2' and Multiple Regression 'R' were applied to test the hypotheses. The level of significance set for testing hypotheses was 0.05.

FINDINGS OF THE STUDY

Demographic Characteristics of Adolescent Girls of Junior Colleges

- ❖ Maximum number i.e. 41.1 per cent in Experimental Group and 39 per cent in Control Group were of 16 years age; 33.3 per cent in Experimental group and 35 per cent in Control Group were of 15 years age and 25.6 per cent in Experimental group and 26 per cent in Control Group were of 17 years old.
- ❖ Around 51.7 per cent in Control Group and 46.7 per cent in Experimental Group were in first year intermediate and 48.3 per cent in Control Group and 53.3 per cent in Experimental Group were in the second year intermediate.
- ❖ As regards to the Group in intermediate first year, 61.29 per cent in control group and 64.29 per cent

in experimental group were studying science group subjects. About 38.71 per cent in control group and 35.71 per cent in experimental group were studying Arts group subjects. In intermediate second year 61 per cent in control group and 62.5 in Experimental Group were studying science group subjects while 39 in control group and 37.5 in experimental group were studying Arts group subjects.

- According to their Area of Residence 42.2 per cent in Control Group and 64.4 per cent in Experimental Group were living in rural area, while 57.8 per cent in Control Group and 35.6 per cent of Experimental Group were living in urban area.
- Majority of the subjects i.e. 63.3 per cent in control group and 58.9 per cent in experimental group were Hindus; 31.7 per cent in Control Group and 37.2 per cent in Experimental Group were Christians and 5 per cent Control Group and 3.9 per cent Experimental Group were Muslims.
- Majority of the sample i.e. 41.6 per cent in Control Group and 52.8 per cent in Experimental Group were Other Caste; 26.7 in Control Group and 30 per cent in Experimental Group were Scheduled Caste; 30 per cent in Control Group and 13.9 per cent in Experimental Group were Backward Caste. while only 1.7 in Control Group and 3.3 per cent in Experimental Group were Scheduled Tribes.
- Majority i.e. 78.3 per cent in Control Group and 78.9 per cent in Experimental Group belonged to Nuclear family, and 16.7 per cent in Control Group and 18.9 per cent in Experimental Group belonged to Joint family, while only 5 per cent in Control Group and 2.2 per cent in Experimental Group belonged to Extended family.
- According to the percentage distribution of the Family's monthly income of the sample 26.1 per cent

in Control Group and 27.8 per cent in Experimental Group had family monthly income between 1001-2000 rupees. About 22.8 per cent in Control Group and 12.2 per cent in Experimental Group had family income between 2001-3000 rupees. A 15 per cent in Control Group and 13.9 in Experimental Group had family monthly income between 4001-5000 rupees, and 15 per cent in Control Group and 13.3 per cent in Experimental Group had family monthly income of rupees 5001 and above, about 13.3 per cent in Control Group and 11.7 per cent in Experimental Group had family monthly income between 3001-4000 rupees. while only 7.8 per cent in control group and 21.1 per cent in experimental group had monthly income of rupees below 1000 rupees.

❖ Majority of the sample i.e.. 97.2 per cent in Control Group and 96.1 per cent in Experimental Group have heard about HIV/AIDS and 2.8 per cent in Control Group and 3.9 per cent in Experimental Group have not heard about HIV/AIDS before this study.

❖ With regard to the sources of knowing about HIV/AIDS, 56.1 per cent of students in control group, 46.1 per cent of students in experimental group came to know about HIV/AIDS through television. Around 32.8 per cent in control group and 21.1 per cent in experimental group came to know from peers. A 22.2 per cent in control group and 24.4 per cent in experimental group indicated news papers as their source of knowing HIV/AIDS. About 20.6 per cent in control group and 25 per cent in experimental group stated that they came to know about HIV/AIDS through health workers. Only 10.6 per cent in control group and 11.7 per cent in experimental group indicated radio as their source of knowing HIV AIDS, and 11.1 per cent in control group and 9.4

per cent in experimental group could know about HIV/AIDS from sign boards posters displayed on the roads and public areas.

- ❖ The sample's responses to a question on "have you ever attended any HIV: AIDS Education Programme before" showed that a 64.4 per cent of students in control group and 67.2 per cent of students in experimental group had not attended any Programme on AIDS, while 35.6 per cent in control group and 32.8 per cent in experimental group had attended AIDS Education Programme.
- ❖ Majority i.e., about 60.9 per cent of students in control group and 59.4 per cent of students in experimental group had attended AIDS Education Programme organised by the government, while 39.1 per cent in control group and 40.6 per cent in experimental group had attended AIDS Education Programme organised by the non-government organisations.
- ❖ The subjects in response to a question "do you feel the need to learn more about HIV/AIDS" stated that they all wanted to know (100%) more about HIV/AIDS.
- ❖ With regard to their knowledge about HIV testing centres it was found that about 85.6 per cent in control group and 84.4 per cent in experimental group did not know where the HIV testing centers are located, while only 12.8 per cent in control group and 15.6 per cent in experimental group stated that they knew the places of HIV testing centres.
- ❖ With regard to HIV/AIDS counselling centres, around 85.6 per cent of students in control group and 86.7 per cent of students in experimental group did not know about the counselling centres, while only 14.4 per cent in control group and 13.8 per cent in experimental group knew the places of counselling centres.

Description of Knowledge, Attitude and Practice Scores of the sample on HIV/AIDS

- The mean Knowledge scores (141.5) of Junior college students belonging to experimental group in post-test I was much higher than their mean pre-test Knowledge scores (97.6). There was no significant difference between mean post-test I Knowledge scores (102) and pre-test Knowledge scores (101.52) of Junior college students belonging to control group.
- The mean percentage of Knowledge scores of junior college students in pre-test and post-test I, show that there was no significant difference found between mean percentages of Control group in pre-test (67.3) and post-test I (68) Knowledge scores, as the gain in Knowledge score was very slight (0.7). Where as in case of the experimental group, the post-test I Knowledge scores increased to 94.35 from 65.08 with a knowledge score gain by 29.27. It indicates that the AEP helped to increase the Knowledge of experimental group on HIV/AIDS.
- The experimental group students' mean post-test I Attitude score (141.19), was higher than their mean pre-test Attitude score (92.81). There was no significant difference found between mean post-test I Attitude score (99.37) and pre-test Attitude scores (99.85) of Junior college students belonging to control group.
- The mean percentage of Attitude scores of students in pre-test and post-test I on HIV/AIDS shows that there was no significant difference between mean percentage of Attitude scores in pre-test (66.25) and post-test 1 (66.57) of control group, and the gain in Attitude scores was also very slight (0.32). Where as in the experimental group the Attitude score in post-test I has increased to 93.51 from 62.10, with a gain of 31.41. It indicates that the AEP helped to bring

a positive change in the Attitude of experimental group regarding HIV/AIDS.

- ❖ The mean post-test I Practice scores (139.60) of Junior college students belonging to experimental group was much higher than their mean pre-test Practice scores (89.42). There was no significant difference between mean pre-test Practice scores (96.43) and post-test I Practice scores (96.87) of Junior college students belonging to control group.
- ❖ The mean percentage scores of Junior college students in pre-test and post-test Practice scores on HIV/AIDS shows that there was no significant difference between mean percentages of pre-test (64.31) and post-test I (64.58). Practice scores of control group and the gain in Practice score was very slight (0.27). Where as in the experimental group the post-test I Practice scores increased to 93.10, from 59.62 with a gain of 33.48. It indicates that the AEP helped to improve healthy Practices in the experimental group regarding HIV/AIDS.
- ❖ The mean Post-test I KAP scores of experimental group (K=141.5, A=140.19, P=139.28) were much higher than the post-test I scores of control group (K=102. A=99.85, P=96.87), indicating the effectiveness of AIDS Education Programme. The pre-test and post-test I KAP scores of control group are almost same indicating that the low score was due to their non-exposure to AIDS Education programme.
- ❖ In the Experimental Group, the pre-test Knowledge scores were in the range of 78 to 118 with a mean of 97.6 and median 97. The post-test I scores were in range of 133 to 148 with a mean of 141.5 and median 141.44. In pre-test and post-test I scores the mean was right to the median. The distribution in pre-test scores were negatively skewed, whereas

the post-test I distribution was more of leptokurtic as the distribution was more peaked than normal distribution. The frequency polygon reveals that the post-test I Knowledge scores were at the higher end of the scale than the pre-test scores which determines the effectiveness of AEP.

- In the Experimental Group the pre-test Attitude scores were in the range of 70 to 119 with a mean of 92.81 and median 91.4. The post-test I scores were in range of 133 to 146 with a mean of 140.19 and median 140.33. The distribution in pre-test scores was negatively skewed, whereas the post-test I distribution was more peaked than normal distribution. The frequency further reveals that the post-test I Attitude scores were at the higher end of the scale than the pre-test scores which determines the effectiveness of AEP.
- In the Experimental Group the pre-test Practice scores were in the range of 70 to 119 with a mean of 89.43 and median 88.1. The post-test I scores were in range of 133 to 145 with a mean of 139.31 and median 139.60. The distribution in pre-test scores was negatively skewed, whereas the post-test I distribution was more peaked than normal distribution. The frequency polygon further reveals that the post-test I Practice scores were at the higher end of the scale than the pre-test scores which determines the effectiveness of AEP.

Effectiveness of AIDS Education Programme in Terms of Difference in Pre-test and Post-test I Knowledge, Attitude and Practice Scores

- There was a significant difference between mean post-test I Knowledge scores (141.52) and mean pre-test Knowledge scores (97.63) in the experimental group. The 't' value was significant at .001 level of significance ('t' = 64.0, P< .001). Hence, null hypothesis HO_1 was rejected and the research hypothesis H, was accepted, indicating that the AEP was significantly effective in increasing the Knowledge of adolescent girls belonging to the experimental group.

❖ The mean pre-test Attitude score was 92.81, and post-test I was 140.19. The 't' value vas significant at .001 level of significance ('t' = 59.77, P< .001). Hence, the null hypothesis HO_2 was rejected and the research hypothesis H_2 was accepted indicating the gain in Attitude was significant and not by chance. This indicates that the AEP was effective in bringing positive change in the Attitude of students belonging the experimental group.

❖ The mean pre-test Practice score was 89.43 and post-test I was 139.29. Whereas the maximum score was 150. The 't' value was significant at .001 level of significance ('t'=56.79, P< .001). Hence, the null hypothesis HO_3 was rejected and the research hypothesis H_3 was accepted indicating the gain in Practice was significant and not by chance. This indicates that the AEP was effective in bringing positive change in the Practice of Junior college students belonging to experimental group.

❖ The actual gain in Knowledge scores (43.89) of Experimental Group was higher than the actual gain (1.17) of Control Group. The modified gain score of Experimental Group (0.84) was significantly higher than the modified gain score of Control Group (0.024). The mean gain score of experimental group was significantly higher than the control group ('t' = 66.50 P < .001). Hence. the null hypothesis (HO_4) was rejected and research hypothesis is (H_4) accepted. In indicates that the AEP was an effective method for enhancing the Knowledge of Junior College Students belonging to experimental group.

- The actual gain of Attitude scores (47.38) of Experimental Group was higher than the actual gain (0.48) of Control Group. The modified gain score of Experimental Group (0.83) was significantly higher than the modified gain score of Control Group (0.0095). This depicts that the Experimental Group's Attitude was higher than the Control Group regarding HIV/AIDS. The mean gain score of sample exposed to AIDS Education Programme was significantly higher than those not exposed to AEP 't' = 74.38 P < .001. Hence, the null hypothesis (HO_5) is rejected and research hypothesis is (H_5) accepted. In indicates that the AEP was an effective method for a favorable Attitude of Junior College Students regarding HIV/AIDS.
- The actual gain of Practice scores (49.86) of Experimental Group was higher than the actual gain (0.44) of Control Group. The modified gain score of Experimental Group (0.82) was significantly higher than the modified gain score of Control Group (0.0082). This depicts that the Experimental Group's Practice was higher than the Control Group regarding HIV/AIDS. The mean gain score of sample exposed to AIDS Education Programme was significantly higher than those not exposed to AEP 't' = 74.38 P <.001. Hence, the null hypothesis (HO_6) was rejected and research hypothesis was (H_6) accepted. In indicates that the AEP was an effective method for a favorable Attitude of Junior College Students regarding HIV/AIDS.

Relationship between Knowledge, Attitude and Practice Scores of Experimental Group Regarding HIV/AIDS before and after AIDS Education Programme

- The correlation between pre-test Knowledge and Attitude scores was 0.836, which is significant at 0.01 level. The correlation between post-test I Knowledge and Attitude score was 0.966, which was also significant at 0.01 level. Hence, the research hypothesis H_7 was accepted and null hypothesis HO_7 was rejected.

- The correlation between pre-test Knowledge and Practice scores was 0.784, which is significant at 0.01 level. The correlation between post-test Knowledge and Practice score was 0.432, which was also significant at 0.01 level. Hence, the research hypothesis H_8 was accepted and null hypothesis HO_8 was rejected.
- The correlation between pre-test Attitude and Practice scores was 0.855, which was significant at 0.01 level. The correlation between post-test I Knowledge and Practice score was 0.587, which was also significant at 0.01 level. Hence, the research hypothesis H_9 was accepted and null hypothesis HO_9 was rejected.
- The correlation between post-test II Knowledge and Attitude was 0.668 and Knowledge and Practice scores was 0.478, which was significant at 0.01 level. The correlation between post-test II Attitude and Practice score was 0.440. which was also significant at 0.01 level. This indicates that the reinforcement of AEP and Peer Group discussion regarding HIV/ AIDS among junior college students was effective in sustaining Knowledge, favourable Attitude and Practice regarding HIV/AIDS. Hence, the research hypothesis H_{10} was accepted and null hypothesis HO_{10} was rejected.
- The correlation between post-test I and post-test II Knowledge, Attitude and Practice scores had positive correlation values significant at 0.01 level. This indicates the AIDS Education Programme and Peer Group discussion regarding HIV/AIDS among junior college students was effective in increasing the Knowledge, a favourable Attitude and Practice.

Hence, the research hypothesis H_{11} was accepted and null hypothesis HO_{11} was rejected.

Association between Independent Variables such as Age, Year of Study in Intermediate, Place of Residence, Religion, Caste, Type of Family, and Income of the family and dependent variables Knowledge, Attitude and Practice

- The Chi-square value (23.13) to establish the association between the Knowledge scores and Age of the sample; X^2 (39.2) between Knowledge scores and year of study: X^2 (38) between Knowledge scores and Place of Residence: X^2 (28.13) between Knowledge scores and Religion; X^2 (15.34) between Knowledge scores and Caste; X^2 (22.16) between Knowledge scores and Type of Family; and X^2 (9.64) between Knowledge scores and Monthly Family Income of Junior college students was found to be statistically significant at 0.05 level. Hence, the null hypothesis was rejected HO_{12} and research hypothesis H_{12} was accepted.
- The Chi-square value (21.95) to establish the association between the Attitude scores and Age of the sample; X^2 (29.81) between Attitude scores and year of study; X^2 (35.95) between Attitude scores and Place of Residence; X^2 (16.64) between Attitude scores and Religion; X^2 (14.99) between Attitude scores and Caste; X^2 (16.89) between Attitude scores and Type of Family; and X^2 (5.92) between Attitude scores and Monthly Family Income of Junior college students was found to be statistically significant at 0.05 level. Hence, the null hypothesis HO_{13} was rejected and research hypothesis H_{13} was accepted.
- The Chi-square value X^2 (25.44) to establish the association between the Age of the sample and Practice scores; X^2 (29.17) between Practice scores and year of study; X^2 (26.58) between Practice scores and Place of Residence; X^2 (18.92) between Practice

scores and Religion; X^2 (13.70) between Practice scores and Caste; X^2 (20.19) between Practice scores and Type of Family; and X^2 (5.64) between Practice scores and Monthly Family Income of Junior college students was found to be statistically significant at 0.05 level. Hence, the null hypothesis HO_{14} was rejected and research hypothesis H_{14} was accepted.

- ❖ The values of Multiple Regression – R^2 values for Experimental group pre-test Knowledge scores and pre-test Attitude scores was R^2 = 0.698 followed by pre-test Practice scores R^2 = 0.717. For post-test I Knowledge scores, post-test Attitude scores was R^2 = 0.564 and post-test Practice scores R^2 = 0.187.
- ❖ The values of Multiple Regression R^2 values for Control Group pre-test Knowledge scores and pre-test Attitude scores was R^2 = 0.519 followed by pre-test Practice scores R^2 = 0.345. For post-test I Knowledge scores and post-test I Attitude scores was R^2 = 0.435 and post-test I Practice scores R^2 = 0. 266. All R^2 values were significant at .0001 level. Thus. null hypothesis HO_{15} was rejected and research hypothesis H_{15} was accepted indicating that there was significant contribution of Knowledge test scores to Attitude and Practice tests scores.

IMPLICATIONS OF THE STUDY

The implications of the study are vital to AIDS education and research.

AIDS Education

Education is an important component of preventing the spread of HIV. There are two main reasons for AIDS education, the first of which is to prevent new infections from taking place. This can be seen as consisting of two processes:

- ❖ Giving people information about HIV-what HIV and AIDS are, how they are transmitted, and how people can protect themselves from infection.

❖ Teaching people how to put this information to use and act on it practically-how to suggest and practice safe sex, how to prevent infection in a medical environment or when injecting drugs.

The second reason people need AIDS education is to reduce stigma and discrimination, in many countries there is a great deal of fear and stigmatisation of people who are HIV positive. Discrimination against positive people can help the AIDS epidemic to spread - if people are fearful of being tested for HIV. and then they are more likely to pass the infection to someone else witout knowing.

AIDS Education can be presented in many ways and put across by many forms of media, which should be selected with the target group in mind. Some people may be best reached by print media while others by video or electronic media. AIDS education needs to embrace culturally appropriate and relevant media.

AIDS education must be based on local resources and needs and must be accepted by the community through their full participation. School and College education curricula should emphasise increasingly on HIV/AIDS and importance of universal precautions in teaching. Teachers need ability to teach adolescents and youth through various teaching strategies. Innovative methods need to be tried out, appropriate and practical strategies may be used to increase awareness, bring about change in attitude and risk behaviour of adolescents and other people in general specially those who are vulnerable. AIDS education must seek to empower youth with confidence, knowledge and skills to prevent the spread of HIV. It must contribute toward a reduction in the transmission of HIV; AIDS through effectively reaching adolescents with reproductive health information and promoting positive attitudes and behaviour.

To achieve the aim of the AIDS education teachers need to be trained to lead the youth and train them in peer education, adolescent sexual and reproductive health issues. These youth can be empowered to disseminate information among their peers to encourage life skills development, communication, and behavour change. This dissemination can take place either on a one-to-one counselling basis or during outreach activities.

Peer education is a social form of education where peers are people form the target group to be educated. Peer education should be an ongoing process and it gives people the opportunity to ask questions outside an academic environment and with someone who isn't an authority figure. Peer education is fond to be most suitable and effective with young people.

Education for promotion of health and prevention of disease is the first of the eight essential components of primary health care. Availability of information regarding prevention and control of HIV/AIDS should be approachable, affordable and acceptable to the people at the cost they can afford and should reflect the concept of primary health care.

The AIDS Education programme model tested as part of the study is found to be very effective in terms of the curriculum, methodology and monitoring. Hence. the replication of the AEP model will be highly effective in Educating adolescents on HIV/AIDS and in the prevention control of HIV/AIDS among them.

AIDS Research

Improvement implies change. The process of change has, in fact, been the subject of a considerable amount of study in recent years. Researchers can act as change agents in motivating community participation in fighting against the AIDS epidemic. Researchers can take up studies on assessing the knowledge, attitude, belief, and practice of people in particular those at risk regarding HIV/AIDS. Change in people can be evaluated by successful implementation of education on AIDS. Research in this field can contribute in the care of those affected by HIV/AIDS and their need for counselling and rehabilitation. Researchers can recommend to the Government and NGOs about the special needs of those affected with HIV/AIDS, and those who are at high risk for infection can be protected.

Research on Comprehensive AIDS Education can greatly contribute to make pupils aware of the need to protect themselves against infection. It can also bring about gradual changes in the wider social environment making safer sex more acceptable. Researchers have tested the effectiveness of an extra-curricular AIDS education programme on schools in rural south east Uganda. After a year they found that the programme was poorly implemented by specially trained teachers and had little over all effect. AIDS Education should be included and examined as part of the national curriculum the study concluded.

A range of different research methods is needed in order to understand the effectiveness of different approaches of AIDS education. Large scale experimental designs may be necessary to identify behavioural change. However, smaller qualitative studies are needed to make sense of these results and to support the development of practice.

There is a growing interest in measuring the effectiveness of different programmes and models of teaching Sex/AIDS education. Such research can guide governments. education and health authorities, advisers, educational institutions. teachers, health care persons and trainers in improving the sex/AIDS education and ensuring it meets the needs of young people. The interest in effectiveness reflects the trends towards evidence based and demonstrable outcomes in education.

If research findings are to be translated into better sex education for young people. then it is essential to disseminate these in ways which are meaningful and accessible to practitioners. This means more than just publication in research reports. academic journals and conference presentations. Opportunities are needed for researcher to join the advisors, trainers and practitioners to share in the interpretation of their work and consider its implications for the future development of AIDS education. This in turn implies a need for closer strategic cooperation between agencies which fund research and agencies which support AIDS education development and training.

CONCLUSION

Based on the findings of the study the following conclusions were drawn:

1. All the subjects were in the Age Group of 15-17 years and were very interested and willing to learn. Thus it may be concluded that these young, energetic, and motivated Adolescent Girls are empowered to develop Knowledge, positive Attitude and healthy Practices regarding HIV/AIDS and have potentialities to spread the message of health and prevent HIV/AIDS among their families and Peer Groups.
2. Innovative AIDS Education Programmes incorporating education material in print and electronic media need to be developed for effectiveness of AIDS education programmes.
3. Adolescent Girls in this study had inadequate Knowledge, Attitude and Practice regarding HIV AIDS. This indicates that they have high learning needs regarding HIV/AIDS. Therefore, there is need to increase the Knowledge. develop positive Attitude and favourable Practice Adolescent Girls by regularly conducting such AIDS Education Programmes and other Health Awareness Programmes, thus tap health care manpower resources from within the community, so that these Young Girls will be able to reach out to the others in the society with AIDS awareness message.
4. The AIDS Education Programme used in this study was found to be effective in increasing the Knowledge, Attitude and Practice on HIV/AIDS. Hence, there is an urgent need to empower the Young Adolescent Girls and Women about HIV/AIDS and other health-related programmes, so that they become active links between the community and the health care delivery system.

5. The AIDS Education Programme along with Peer Group discussion was found to be effective method of providing information to Adolescent Girls and regarding HIV/AIDS. This indicates such health awareness programmes need to be conducted to bring change in the people especially in those high-risk groups like Women, Adolescents and Children. Further it indicates that the Adolescent Girls need more than one teaching or a combination of different methods of learning e.g. Peer Group teaching or discussion to gain maximum Knowledge, Attitude and Practice on HIV/AIDS. This also indicates that there is a need for using various innovative strategies to bring not only awareness but also change in Attitude and risk behaviour of vulnerable among high risk Groups like Women, Youth and Children.

RECOMMENDATIONS

The following recommendations are made based on the present study:

1. Replication of the same study on a large sample may help to draw conclusions that are more definite and generalise to a larger population.

2. A comparative study may be conducted on both Adolescent Boys and Girls from high schools and junior colleges.

3. A study may be conducted using self-instructional module for health care personnel like nursing staff. student nurses, lab technicians and other health care personnel on their Knowledge, Attitude and Practices in health care settings.

4. A case study may be carried out on quality of life of persons with HIV infection/AIDS.

5. Replication of AIDS Education programme model and the methodology of the present study may be carried out for effective AIDS education to adolescents.

References

1. Abdella, F.G., and Levine, E. 1979. Better Patient Care through Nursing Research. New York: Mac Millan.

2. Aggarwal., and Kumar. 1996. Awareness of AIDS Among School Children in Haryana. *Indian Journal of Public Health* 40(2) 38-45.

3. Agha, S., and Rossem, R. 2004. Impact of a School-based Peer Sexual Health Intervention on Normative Beliefs, Risk Perceptions, and Sexual Behaviour of Zambian Adolescents. *Journal of Adolescent Health* 34 (5) 441-452.

4. Aplasca., Siegel., Madel., Paul., Monzon., and Hearst. 1995. Results of a Model AIDS Prevention Programme for High School Students in Philippines. AIDS Supplement 1, 7-13.

5. AP AIDS Control Project. 1995. HIV/AIDS and Women. Government of Andhra Pradesh, Hyderabad.

6. AP State AIDS Control Society. 2005. HIV/AIDS in Andhra Pradesh Situation and Response: A Report 2005.

7. AP State AIDS Control Society. 2004. Break the Silence—Talk about AIDS. Current Scenario of HIV/AIDS in Andhra Pradesh, Hyderabad.

8. AIDS Action. 1994. The International Newsletter on AIDS Prevention and Care 25, 4-5.

9. Awasthi, S., Nichter, M., and Pande, V.K. 2000. Developing an interactive STD-prevention Programme for Youth; Lessons from a North Indian Slum. Studies in Family Planning 31, 138-150.

10. Babola., Sakolsky., Vondrasek., Mounlom., and Tchupo. 2001. The Impact of a Community Mobilisation Project on Health Related Knowledge and Practices in Camaroon. Journal of Community Health 26. 459-477.

11. Bajaj. 1993. *A Study to Evaluate the Effectiveness of Self-Instructional Module on AIDS, Its Prevention and Control in Terms of Knowledge of Third Year General Nursing Students.*. Unpublished M.N Thesis. University of Delhi.

12. Barua. 1996. *A Study to Assess the Knowledge of Anganwadi Workers Nutrition of Under Five Children, with a View to Prepare a Health Education Programme on Nutrition of the Children 0-5 for the Anganwadi Workers in a Selected Area of Delhi.* Unpublished MN Thesis, University of Delhi.

13. Basset, M., and Sherman, J. 1994. Female Sexual Behaviour and the Risk of HIV Infection: An Ethnographic Study in Harare, Zimbabwe. Women and AIDS Programme Research Reports Series. Washington DC: International Center for Research on Women.

14. Best, W. J., and Kahn, V.J. 1992. Research in Education 6th ed. New Delhi: Prentice Hall of India.

15. Bhaduri, A., and Farell, N. 1981. Health Research A Community Based Approach, New Delhi: W.H.O Regional Office for South East Asia.

16. Birru. 1997. A *Study to Evaluate the effectiveness of Planned Teaching Progrannne for Commercial Sex Workers Regarding Prevention and Control of HIV/AIDS in a Selected District of Maharastra.* Unpublished MN Thesis, University of Delhi.

17. Baggaley., R. 1996. Young People Talk about HIV: Summary of Findings from 45 Focus Group Discussions Carried Out With Young People from Youth Groups and Schools. Lusaka: UNICEF.

18. Bhuiya., Hanifi., Hossain., and Aziz. 2000. Effects of an AIDS Awareness Campaign on Knowledge about AIDS in a Remote Rural Area in Bangladesh. International Health Education, 19, 51-63.

19. Bosompra. 1992. The Potential of Drama and Songs as Channels for AIDS Education in Africa: A Report on Focus Group Findings from Ghana. International Quarterly of Community Health Education 12, 317-342.

20. Burns N., and Grove, K. 1999. The Practice of Nursing Research 3rd edition, London: W.B. Saunders Company.

21. Cain., Richard., Schulze., Rick., Preston., and Deborah. 2001. Developing a Partnership for HIV Primary Prevention for Men

at High Risk for HIV Infection in Rural Communities. International Journal of Health Promotion and Education 32, 45-51.

22. Centers for Disease Control and Prevention. 1998. Youth Risk Behaviour Survey 1997, Altanta.

23. CHAI. 1995. Policy and Plan of Action on HIV Infection and AIDS. Secunderabad. Catholic Health Association of India.

24. CHARCA. 2005. The New Campaign, "Commitment to Protect the Young and Vulnerable," International Women's Day, March 8, 2004.

25. Chaterjee., Misra., and Rao. 2003. Indian Health Report 2003. New Delhi. Oxford University Press.

26. Chaturvedi., Gupta., Rajoura., Kumar., and Aggarwal. 1999. Impact of a Multi-promotional Package on Awareness and Knowledge about STD and AIDS Among the Trainees of an Industrial Training Institute in a Resettlement Colony of Delhi, India, Journal Communicable Diseases, 31(4), 209-216.

27. C.H.E.B. 1998. AIDS Information for Health Care Workers for Protection Against AIDS. Central Health Education Bureau, New Delhi.

28. Christian Medical Commission. 1987. What is AIDS?—A Manual for Health Workers. Geneva: World Council of Churches.

29. Collins and Rau. 2000. Prevention of AIDS in the World: A Global Report. Edited by Mann J. Harvard College.

30. Daniel, 1995. A Study to Develop and Determine the Effectiveness of the Self-instructional Module on HIV/AIDS Prevention and Control for Multipurpose Health Workers Based on their Identified Learning Needs in Selected District in Rajasthan. Unpublished MN Thesis. University of Delhi.

31. Dark., Gates., Holley., Malunga., and Arnold. (1990). Rapid KABP Survey for evaluation of NGO HIV/AIDS Prevention Projects. AIDS Education and Prevention 8, 143-154.

32. Dhasaradhan. Indrani. 2001. A Study to Assess the Knowledge and Attitude of Nurses Towards HIV/AIDS Patients in Chennai. Nursing Journal of India 52 (12) 273-274.

33. Dutta. 1993. A Study on the Impact of Awareness Programme Imparted to In-service Nursing Staff on their Knowledge Regarding AIDS. Indian Journal of Public Health 37 (1) 23-25.

34. Elkins., Maticka., Kiewying., Chantapreeda., Sommapat., and Theerasobhon. 1996. Evaluation of HIV/AIDS Education Initiative among Women in North-Eastern Thai Villages, Journal of Tropical Medical Public Health 27. 430-442.

35. FAGans., and Hope. (1998). Promoting Behaviour Change: An Assessment of the Peer Education HIV/AIDS Prevention Programme at the Workplace. Journal of Health Communication, 8 267-281.

36. Fitgerad., and Stanton. (1999). An Evaluatin of an Education Programme by HIV Infection Suing Puppetry. AIDS Care 3(3), 317-329.

37. Flaskerud, H.J. 1989. AIDS/HIV Infection A Reference Guide for Nursing Professionals, Philadelphia: W.B. Saunders Company.

38. Family Health International. 1996. Let Their Voices Be Heard: Empowering Women in the Fight Against. AIDS, Volume II, No 3, May 1996.

39. Gaitonde, Ishwas R. 2001. A Thief in the Night: Understanding AIDS. East West Books, Chennai.

40. Garg. 1994. Information, Education and Communication in AIDS Prevention. Swasth Hind Nov-Dec. 1994.

41. Garrett, H. E., and Woodsworth, R.S. 1981. Statistics in Psychology and Education. Bombay: Vakils Feffer and Simon Ltd.

42. Gilbert, J.J. 1983. Educational Handbook for Health Personnel. Geneva: WHO.

43. Government of A-P, APSACS, APARD, UNICEF. 2004. HIV/AIDS young People Initiative in Schools a Workbook for Teachers in Secondary Schools of Andhra Pradesh.

44. Handa. 1994. A *Study to Identify the Learning Needs of High School Students on Human Sexuality with a View to Develop and Evaluate the Effectiveness of a Sex Education Programme in Public Schools of South Delhi.* Trained Nurses Association of India, Nursing Year Book 2000.

45. Halewood., and Kenny. 2006. An Evaluation of HIV Prevention Programme. AIDS Education and Prevention 11, 203-211.

46. Hindustan Times. 2006. Report about HIV Positive Woman is Running for Legislature in India's Assam State.

47. Human Development Report. 2000. Published by Oxford University Press, New Delhi.

48. Jimmott, J.B., and Jemmott, L.S. 1994. Interventions for Adolescents in Community Settings, Preventing AIDS: Theories and Methods of Behavioural Interventions. New York.

49. Jimmott, J.B., Jemmott, L.S., and Fong, G.T. 1998. Abstinence and Safer Sex HIV Risk Reduction Interventions for African American Adolescents: A Randomised Controlled Trial. Journal of the American Medial Association. 27. 1529-1536.

50. Kagimu., Marum., Nakyanjo., Walakira., and Hogle. 1998. Evaluation of the Effectiveness of AIDS Health Education Intervention in the Muslim Community in Uganda. AIDS Education and Prevention 10(3) 215-228.

51. Kalpana. 2001. Playing Ostrich with AIDS; The Debate Over Numbers is Futile, Times of India, 12th June 2001.

52. Kasule. 1997. Zimbabwean Teenagers' Knowledge of AIDS and Other Sexually Transmitted Diseases. East Africa Medical Journal, 74:76-81.

53. Kerlinger, F.N. 1973. Foundations of Behavioural Research, New York: Holt International.

54. Kinsman., and Whitworth. 2001. Evaluation of a Comprehensive School-based AIDS Education Programme in Rural Makasa, Uganda. Health Education Research.

55. Klepp., Ndeki., Seha., Hannan., Msuya., Irema., and Schreiner. 1994. AIDS Education for Primary School Children in Tanzania: an Evaluation Study. AIDS: 1157-1162.

56. Koichiro Matsuura. 2004. UNESCO, International Women's Day, 8 March 2004.

57. Krauss, B.J., Godfrey, C.. and Yee, D. 2000. Saving our Children from a Silent Epidemic: The Path Programme for Parents and Preadolescents. Sage Publications, Thousand Oaks, pp. 89-112.

58. Kuhn., Steinberg., and Mathews. 1994. Participation of the School Community in AIDS Education: An Evaluation of a High School Programme in South Africa. AIDS Care, 6(2), 161-171.

59. Kumar., Mehra., Singh., Badhan., and Gulati. 1995. Teachers Awareness and Opinion about AIDS: Implications for School Based AIDS Education. Journal of Communicable Diseases 27(2), 101-106.

60. Kurian. 1998. A Comparative Study to Assess the Effectiveness of Planned Teaching Programme Regarding Adolescent Reproductive Health on Knowledge, Attitude and Practice of High School Girls in Selected Urban and Rural High Schools of Kerala. Unpublished M.N Thesis, University of Delhi.

61. International Federation of Red Cross. 1992. Caring for People with AIDS at Home. Geneva: Red Cross and Red Crescent Societies.

62. Lema, V.M., and Hassan, MA. 1994. Knowledge of Sexually Transmitted Diseases. HIV Infection and AIDS Among Sexually Active Adolescents in Nairobi. Kenya and its Relationship to their Sexual Behaviour and Contraception. East Africa Med. Journal 71:122-128.

63. Majumdar., and Roberts. 1998. AIDS Awareness among Women: The Benefit of Culturally Sensitive Educational Programmes,. International Journal of Health Care of Women 19(2), 141-153.

64. Maswanya., Moji., Aoyagi., Yahata., Kusano., and Nagata. 2000. Knowledge and Attitudes Toward AIDS among Female College Students in Nagsaki, Japan. Health Education and Research 15, 15-11.

65. Matasha E. 1998. Sexual and Reproductive Health Among Primary and Secondary School Pupils in Mwanza, Tanzania: Need for Intervention. AIDS Care, 10: 571-82.

66. Maticka., Elkins., Kuyyakanond., and Kiewying. 1994, A Research-Based HIV Intervention in Thailand. Health Transition Review. 4, 349-367,

67. Matthews, C., Ellison, G., Guttmacher, S., (1999), Can Audio-visual Presentation be Used to Provide Health Education at Primary Care Facilities in South Africa. Health. Education Journal 58, 146-156.

68. McGranth, D., and Joseph, W.D. (1999), An HIV/AIDS Awareness and Prevention: Evaluation of Drama and Flyer Distribution Intervention. International Quarterly of Communication Health 16, 237-255.

69. McKusick. 1990. AIDS Behavioural Research Project. American Journal of Public Health 80 (8) 978-83,

70. Meerkers., Stallworth., and Harris, 1997. Changing Adolescent's Beliefs about Protective Sexual Behaviour: PSI Research Division

Working Paper No. 16, Washington: Population Services International.

71. Migliori., Spanevello., Manfrin., Abongomera., Pedretti., and Borghesi. 1996. AIDS and T.B Control Programme: An Integrated Approach at Educational Level. Journal of Chest Diseases, 51(2), 102-107.

72. Miller, B.C., Norti, M.C., and Schavaneveldt, P. 1998. The Timing of Sexual Intercourse among Adolescents: Family, Peer and Other Antecedents. Youth and Society, 29(3), 390.

73. Mitrani., Szapocznik., and Baptista. 2000. Working with Families in the Era of HIV/AID. Sage Publications, New Delhi 243-250.

74. Mohanraj. 2001. India's Response to HIV/AIDS. Herald of Health, Sep., 2001.

75. Mukherje. 1996. AIDS in Women A Tragedy, Your Health, India.

76. Muniammal. 1994. A *Study to Evaluate the Effectiveness* of *Planned Teaching Programme Based on the Learning Needs of Traditional Birth Attendants Regarding Prevention and Control of AIDS in a Selected District* of *Tamilnadu.* Unpublished M.N. Thesis, University of Delhi.

77. Mutatkar. (1998). Towards Reducing the Spread of HIV in Thai Villages: Evaluation of a Village Based Intervention. AIDS Education and Prevention 9(1), 49-69.

78. National AIDS Control Programme India: Country Scenario Update. 1995. NACO, Ministry of Health and Family Welfare, Government of India.

79. NACO Specialist's Training and Reference Module. 1999. Ministry of Health and Family Welfare. Government of India.

80. NACO. 2000. Prime Minister's Meeting with the Business Leaders of India on HIV/AIDS. December 1st 2000—A Press Release.

81. NACO. 1995. HIV Infection/AIDS: Prevention and Control Self-Instructional and Teaching Modules for Pre-Service and In-Service Nurses and Midwives, Ministry of Health and Family Welfare. Government of India.

82. NACO. 2000. What is AIDS, Ministry of Health and Family Welfare. Government of India.

83. NACO. 2000. Training Module for Nurses. New Delhi.

84. NACO. 2004. Programme Implementation Guidelines for a Phased Scale up of Access to Antiretroviral Therapy for People Living with HIV/AIDS.

85. NACO. 2005. HIV AIDS in Andhra Pradesh Situation and Response A Report 2005.

86. NACO. 2005. Observed HIV Prevalence Levels State-wise: 1998-2004.

87. NACO. 2005. Monthly Updates on AIDS, 31 May, 2005.

88. NACO. 2005. HIV Estimates—2004, NACO, 2005.

89. NACO, NCERT. UNICEF, UNESCO. 2000. Learning for Life. A Guide to Family Health and Life Skills Education for Teachers and Students.

90. Ndlovu., and Sihlangu. 1992. Evaluating a School Based Intervention for STD/AIDS Prevention. Journal of Adolescent Health 15, 582-591.

91. Oakley A., Fullerton D. and Holland J. 2002. Sexual Health Education Interventions for Young People. A Methodological Review. British Medical Journal 310:158-62.

92. Parker. 1996. Employment, Community Mobilisation and Social Change in the Face of HIV/AIDS. Journal of Adolescent Health 13, 45-56.

93. Peaqegnat, W., and Bray, J. 1997. Families and HIV/AIDS, Journal of Family Psychology, 11 (1) 3-10.

94. Peersman. 1998. Focus and Effectiveness of HIV Prevention Efforts for Young People. AIDS 12 191-196.

95. Perugu, and Rivo. 1992. Racial Differences in AIDS Knowledge Among Adults. AIDS Education Preview 4(1) 52-60.

96. Pratt. R. 1995. HIV and AIDS A Strategy for Nursing Care. 4th ed. London: J.W. Arrowsmith Ltd.

97. Petro-Nustas and Wasileh. 2000. University Students Knowledge of AIDS. International Journal of Nursing Studies 37, 423-433.

98. Pietrow., Mechalan., Chimombo and Mpemba. (1997). AIDS Education for Youth through Active Learning. International Journal of Educational Development 17, 41-50.

99. Plummer F.A., Simonsen N.J. and Cameron D.W. 1991. Cofactors in Male-female Sexual Transmission of Human Immunodeficiency Virus Type 1. Journal Infectious Diseases 163, 223-39.

100. Polit. F. D., and Hungler, P.B. 1999. Nursing Research Principles and Methods. 6th ed. New York: Lippincott.

101. Puttineni Agostina. 2002. Walk Along with me in an AIDS Free World. Vijayawada, AP India.

102. Ray., Saha., Mandal., Biswas., Dasgupta., and Kumar. 1995. An Assessment of AIDS Awareness Programme for I.C.D.S. Functionaries. Indian Journal of Public Health 39(3), 100-104.

103. Rapkin., Murphy and Munoz. 2000. The Family Health Project: Working with Families in the era of HIV/AIDS. Sage Publications, Thousand Oaks, 231- 242.

104. Ray, G.L. and Mondal, S. 1999. Research Methods in Social Sciences and Extension Education. Published by Nayaprakash Publishers, Calcutta.

105. Richard Levin. I. and David Rubbin, S. 1999. Statistics for Management. Published by Prentice Hall India Private Limited, 7th Edition, New Delhi.

106. Robertson and Leuten (1998). Entertainment Education and HIV/AIDS prevention: A Field Experiment. Journal of Health Communication 5, 81-100.

107. Rodwell, M. 1996. An Analysis of the Concept of Empowerment. Journal of Advanced Nursing 23, 305-313.

108. Rossan., and Meekers. 1999. An Evaluation of the Effectiveness of Targeted Social Marketing to Promote Adolescent and Young Adult Reproductive Health in Camaeron. AIDS Education and Prevention 12, 383-404.

109. Rotary Club of Bhagyanagar and R.C.B. Service Trust. 1998. Crusade Against AIDS, Hyderabad, India.

110. Rubeena, S.D. 1998. The Effect of a Structured Teaching Programme on Breast Cancer and Breast Self Examination BSE in Selected Unmarried Women of Kerala, Master of Philosophy Dissertation, University of MAHE, Manipal.

111. Solidarity and Action Against the HIV Infections in India (SAATHI). 2004, A Directory of HIV/AIDS Services in India.

112. SAKHI. 2000. Solidarity and Action Against the HIV Infections in India: An Intervention Project Among Sex Workers in the North East India. Assam State AIDS Control Society.

113. Sankaranarayana., Naik., Gurunani., Ganesh., Gandewar., Singh., and Vermund. 1996. Impact of School Based HIV/AIDS Education for Adolescents in Bombay, India. Journal Tropical Medial and Public Health 27 (4) 692-695,

114. Schopper., Ayiga., Ezatirale., Idro., and Homsy. 1995. Village Based AIDS Prevention in a Rural District in Uganda, Health Policy and Planning 2, 171-180.

115. Sharma, S.R. 1994. Statistical Methods in Educational Research, Anmol Publications, 1st Edition, New Delhi.

116. Shuey., Babishangire., Omiat., and Bagarukayo. 1999, Increased Sexual Abstinence Among in School Adolescents as a Result of School Health Education in Soroti District, Uganda. Health Education Research: Theory and Practice 14, 411-419.

117. Siddarth, Dube. 2001. Fact and Fiction About AIDS. Times of India, 5th Dec 2001.

118. Simooya., and Sanjobon. 2001. In But Free: An AIDS Intervention in an African Prison, AIDS Education and Prevention 13 (2) 120-130

119. Singer., and Weeks. 1996. Results of a Model AIDS Prevention Programme for High School Students in the Philippines. Journal of Adolescent Health 9. 7-13.

120. Singhal., Aravind., and Rogers. 2003. Combating AIDS: Communication Strategies in Action, Sage Publications, New Delhi.

121. Singh, Sunita. 2001, KAP Study on HIV/AIDS Among Nursing Graduates. Nursing Journal of India, 52 (12) 275-276.

122. Squire, Corinne. 1995. Women and AIDS: Psychological Perspectives. SAGE Publications, New Delhi pp. 73-74, 107-108, 165.

123. Srinivasan. 2000. All You Wanted to Know About HIV and AIDS, New Delhi: Sterling Publications.

124, Srivastava. 1992. AIDS Awareness Amongst School Teachers in a Rural Area of India. Asian Journal of Public Health 6(1), 16-17.

125. Talbot, L.A. 1995, Principals and Practice of Nursing Research, Chicago: C.V. Mosby 317-370.

126. Times of India. 1998. Education Material Titled "AIDS Concerns All" in Collaboration with UNICEF and SCERT.

127. The Bill and Melinda Gates Foundation's Avahan Programme. 2004.

128. The New Indian Express. March 3rd 2006. Report on: Coordinated HIV/AIDS Response Through Capacity Building and Awareness.

129. Todankar., and Sumati. 2000. Impact of School Based HIV and AIDS Education for Adolescents in India. Journal of Public Health, 27(4), 692-695.

130. Treece and Treece. 1986. Essentials of Research in Nursing, St. Louis: The C.V. Mosby Co.

131. UNAIDS/WHO: AIDS Epidemic Update, December 2005.

132. UNAIDS/WHO: Report on the Global AIDS Epidemic Update February 9, 2006.

133. UNAIDS/WHO Epidemiological Fact Sheets on HIV/AIDS and Sexually Transmitted Infections, 2004 Update, India.

134. UNAIDS, AIDS Epidemic Update, December 2006.

135. UNAIDS, AIDS Epidemic Update, December 2005.

136. UNAIDS, AIDS Epidemic Update, December 2004.

137. UNAIDS, AIDS Epidemic Update, December 2003.

138. UNAIDS, HIV and AIDS-related Stigmatisation, Discrimination and Denial: Forms, Contexts and Determinants, June 2000.

139. UNAIDS/India: HIV and AIDS-related Stigmatisation, Discrimination and Denial, August 2001.

140. UNAIDS/WHO. 2004. Epidemiological Fact Sheets on HIV/AIDS and Sexually Transmitted Infections, 2004 Update, India.

141. Valente, T.W., and Bharat, U. (1999). An Evaluation of the Use of Drama to Communicate HIV/AIDS Information. AIDS Education and Prevention. 11, 203-211.

142. Vati, Jogindra., Walia. Indragit., and Sharma, Santosh. 2003. Nursing Journal of India. 54(12) 276-277.

143. Vaughan, P. W., Regis, A., and St Catherine, E. (2000). Effects of an Education Radio Programme on Family Planning and HIV Prevention. International Family Planning Perspectives 26. 148-157.

144. Voluntary Health Association of India (VHAI). 1998. HIV/AIDS for Everybody to Know.

145. Visser, M. 1996. Evaluation of the First AIDS Kit, the AIDS and Life Style Education Programme for Teenagers. South African Journal of Psychology 26, 103-113.

146. World Health Organisation. 1991. AIDS Prevention Through Health Promotion. New Delhi: B.I. Churchill Livingstone.

147. World Health Organisation. 1999. National AIDS Programme Management. Geneva.

148. World Health Organisation. 1995. Information, Education and Communication—A Guide for Programme Managers, New Delhi; Southeast Asia Region.

149. World Development Report. 2007. Development and Next Generation. Published by the World Bank, Washington 31-32, 94-95, 123-124. 131.

150. World Health Organisation. 1996. Handbook on AIDS Home Care. New Delhi. Regional Office of the South East Asia.

151. World Health Organisation. 1997. AIDS: No Time For Complacency. New Delhi. Regional Office for Southeast Asia.

152. World Health Organisation. 1998. AIDS in the Southeast Asia Region, New Delhi: Regional Office for Southeast Asia.

153. World Health Report. 1998. W.H.O., Geneva, Switzerland.

154. World Health Organisation, World AIDS Day I December 2005, SEARO, New Delhi.

155. World Health Organisation. 2000. Let' Talk about AIDS, SEARO, New Delhi.

156. World Health Organisation. 2000. Women and HIV/AIDS, WHO, Geneva.

157. World Health Organisation, World AIDS Day I December 2004, SEARO, New Delhi.

158. World Bank. 2004. World Development Report 2004. Making Services Work for Poor People. Washington: The World Bank and Oxford University Press.

159. World Health Organisation. 2002. HIV/AIDS Strategic Framework for WHO Southeast Asia Region 2002-2006. SEARO, New Delhi.

160. WHO SEARO. (1985). Technical Publications No: 6 Systems Model.

Web Sites

1. www.eldis.org: Articles Related to Research on AIDS Education.
2. www.avert.org/aidseducation.html: NACO, NCERT, UNICEF, UNESCO. 2000. Learning for Life; A Guide to Family Health and Life Skills Education for Teachers and Students.
3. www.developmentgateway.org/youth: AIDS Study and Teaching Youth and Adolescents
4. www.medflash.org.uk: AIDS Research and Education
5. www.nacoindia.org: NACO. 2005. HIV Estimates—2004 NACO, 2005 NACO, and 2006 NACO.
6. www.unaids.ora: UNAIDS WHO; Report on the Global AIDS Epidemic Update February 9. 2006
7. www.un.org/youth: Interventions to Control AIDS and Sexually Transmitted Diseases.
8. www.unicef.org/life Skills; Research Studies on HIV/AIDS Education.
9. www.who.org/child-adolescent-health: Department of Child and Adolescent Health of the World Health Organisation.
10. www.worldbank.org/children/youth: Effects of AIDS Education on Children and Youth.
11. www.worldaidscampaign.org Information and Updates from World AIDS Campaign.
12. www.youandaids.org: Health Education of HIV/AIDS for Prevention Among Adolescents.
13. www.youththink.org: AIDS Education and Counselling
14. www.idrc.ca/en/ev.html: AIDS Counselling and Education: International Development Research Centre.
15. www.caps.ucsf.edu/projects.html: Collaborative HIV/AIDS Prevention Research in Developing Countries.

Index

N

O

P

R

❑❑❑